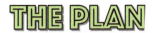

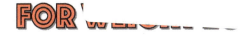

2 Books in 1: Cookbook for Beginners: 240+ Vegetarian and Vegan Recipes to Energize Your Body and Get to Know About How this Diet Can Help to Lose Weight!

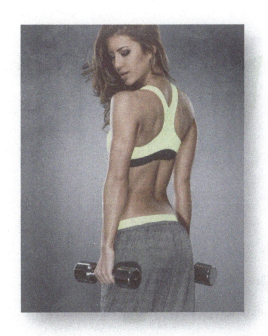

By

Audrey Pottery

TABLE OF CONTENT

PART 1-INTRODUCTION TO THE PLANT-BASED DIET 15

THE BENEFITS OF THE PLANT-BASED DIET 17

HOW TO START TO LOSE WEIGHT 18

THE FUNDAMENTAL FACTORS FOR BEING FIT 20

Breakfast 21

1) Kid-Friendly Cereal 22
2) Original Breakfast Burrito 22
3) Homemade Toast Crunch 22
4) Cinnamon and Apple Oatmeal Cups 22
5) Chickpea Tofu Scramble with Spicy Vegetables 23
6) Coconut Prunes Granola 23
7) Thyme Pumpkin Fry 23
8) Almond Raspberry Smoothie 23
9) Kiwi Oatmeal Bars 24
10) Apple Spicy Pancakes 24
11) Almond and Coconut Granola with Cherries 24
12) Almonds Cinnamon Buckwheat 24
13) Yellow Smoothie 25
14) Hearty Smoothie 25
15) Carrot and Strawberry Smoothie 25
16) Super Green Smoothie 25
17) Blueberry Maple Smoothie 25
18) Power Chia-Peach Smoothie 26
19) PORRIDGE WITH STRAWBERRIES AND COCONUT 26
20) Broccoli Browns 26

Soups, Stew, and Salads 27

21) Roasted Carrot Soup 28
22) Italian Penne Pasta Salad 28
23) Chana Chaat Indian Salad 28
24) Tempeh and Noodle Salad Thai-Style 29
25) Typical Cream of Broccoli Soup 29
26) Raisin Moroccan Lentil Salad 29
27) Chickpea and Asparagus Salad 30
28) Old-Fashioned Green Bean Salad 30
29) Winter Bean Soup 30
30) Italian-Style Cream Mushrooms Soup 31
31) Roasted Basil and Tomato Soup 31
32) Under Pressure Cooker Green Onion and Potato Soup 31
33) Bell Pepper and Mushroom Soup 31
34) Pumpkin Cayenne Soup 32
35) Zucchini Cream Soup with Walnuts 32
36) Ramen Soup 32
37) Black-Eyed Pea Soup 32

Vegetables and Side Dishes 33

38) Roasted Kohlrabi 34
39) Cauliflower with Tahini Sauce 34
40) Herb Cauliflower Mash 34
41) Garlic and Herb Mushroom Skillet 34
42) Pan-Fried Asparagus 35
43) Gingery Carrot Mash 35
44) Mediterranean-Style Roasted Artichokes 35
45) Thai-Style Braised Kale 35

46)	Silky Kohlrabi Puree	36
47)	Creamy Sautéed Spinach	36
48)	Roasted Carrots with Herbs	36
49)	Braised Green Beans	36

Lunch 37

50)	Jalapeño Quinoa Bowl with Lima Beans	38
51)	Avocado Coconut Pie	38
52)	Green Avocado Carbonara	38
53)	Mushroom and Green Bean Biryani	39
54)	Mushroom Lettuce Wraps	39
55)	Classic Garlicky Rice	39
56)	Brown Rice with Vegetables and Tofu	39
57)	Amaranth Porridge	40
58)	Mum's Aromatic Rice	40
59)	Everyday Savory Grits	40
60)	Greek-Style Barley Salad	40
61)	Sweet Maize Meal Porridge	41
62)	Focaccia with Mixed Mushrooms	41
63)	Seitan Cakes with Broccoli Mash	41
64)	Spicy Cheese with Tofu Balls	41
65)	Quinoa and Veggie Burgers	42
66)	Baked Tofu with Roasted Peppers	42
67)	Zoodle Bolognese	42
68)	Zucchini Boats with Vegan Cheese	43
69)	Roasted Butternut Squash with Chimichurri	43
70)	Black Bean Burgers with BBQ Sauce	43

71)	Creamy Brussels Sprouts Bake	43
72)	Baked Cheesy Spaghetti Squash	44
73)	Kale and Mushroom Pierogis	44
74)	Vegan Mushroom Pizza	44

Dinner ... 45

75)	Parsley Carrots and Parsnips	46
76)	Sesame Roasted Broccoli with Brown Rice	46
77)	Matcha-Infused Tofu Rice	46
78)	Chinese Fried Rice	46
79)	Peppered Pinto Beans	47
80)	Black-Eyed Peas with Sun-Dried Tomatoes	47
81)	Vegetarian Quinoa Curry	47
82)	Alfredo Rice with Green Beans	47
83)	Korean-Style Millet	47
84)	Lemony Chickpeas with Kale	48
85)	Dinner Rice and Lentils	48
86)	Sesame Kale Slaw	48
87)	Spicy Steamed Broccoli	48
88)	Garlic Roasted Carrots	48
89)	Eggplant and Hummus Pizza	49
90)	Miso Green Cabbage	49
91)	Steamed Broccoli with Hazelnuts	49
92)	Cilantro Okra	49
93)	Citrus Asparagus	49

Snacks ... 50

94)	Sesame Cabbage Sauté	51

95)	Tomatoes Stuffed with Chickpeas and Quinoa	51
96)	Herbed Vegetable Traybake	51
97)	Louisiana-Style Sweet Potato Chips	51
98)	Bell Pepper and Seitan Balls	52
99)	Parmesan Broccoli Tots	52
100)	Chocolate Bars with Walnuts	52
101)	Carrot Energy Balls	52
102)	Crunchy Sweet Potato Bites	53
103)	Roasted Glazed Baby Carrots	53
104)	Oven-Baked Kale Chips	53
105)	Cheesy Cashew Dip	53
106)	Peppery Hummus Dip	54
107)	Traditional Lebanese Mutabal	54
108)	Indian-Style Roasted Chickpeas	54
109)	Avocado with Tahini Sauce	54

Desserts 55

110)	Chocolate Dream Balls	56
111)	Last-Minute Macaroons	56
112)		56
113)	Old-Fashioned Ratafias	56
114)	Jasmine Rice Pudding with Dried Apricots	56
115)	Chocolate Fudge with Nuts	57
116)	Chocolate and Peanut Butter Cookies	57
117)	Mixed Berry Yogurt Ice Pops	57
118)	Holiday Pecan Tart	57
119)	Coconut Chocolate Barks	58

120)	Nutty Date Cake	58
121)	Berry Cupcakes with Cashew Cheese Icing	58
122)	Coconut and Chocolate Cake	58
123)	Berry Macedonia with Mint	59
124)	Cinnamon Pumpkin Pie	59
125)	Party Matcha and Hazelnut Cheesecake	59

PART 2- INTRODUCTION to PLANT-BASED DIET 69

FOOD TO AVOID 71

BREAKFAST 73

126)	Banana Pancakes	74
127)	Pesto Bread	74
128)	Classic French Toasts	74
129)	Creamy Bread with Sesame	75
130)	Different Seeds Bread	75
131)	Naan Bread	76
132)	Mushroom and Spinach Chickpea Omelette	76
133)	Coconut-Raspberry Pancakes	77
134)	Blueberry-Chia Pudding	77
135)	Potato and Cauliflower Browns	78
136)	Pistachios-Pumpkin Cake	79
137)	Bell Pepper with Scrambled Tofu	79
138)	Original French Toast	80
139)	Frybread with Peanut Butter and Jam	80
140)	Pudding with Sultanas on Ciabatta Bread	81
141)	Vegan Banh Mi	81
142)	Breakfast Nutty Oatmeal Muffins	81

143)	Smoothie Bowl of Raspberry and Chia	82
144)	Breakfast Oats with Walnuts and Currants	82
145)	Applesauce Pancakes with Coconut	82
146)	Veggie Panini	83
147)	Cheddar Grits and Soy Chorizo	84
148)	Vanilla Crepes and Berry Cream Compote Topping	84
149)	Strawberry and Pecan Breakfast	85
150)	Granola with Hazelnuts and Orange	85
151)	Orange Crepes	86
152)	Oat Bread with Coconut	86
153)	Bowl with Black Beans and Spicy Quinoa	86
154)	Almond and Raisin Granola	87
155)	Pecan and Pumpkin Seed Oat Jars	87
156)	Easy Apple Muffins	87
157)	Almond Yogurt with Berries and Walnuts	88
158)	Breakfast Blueberry Muesli	88
159)	Berry and Almond Butter Swirl Bowl	89
160)	Oats with Coconut and Strawberries	89

SOUPS, STEW, AND SALADS 90

161)	Black Bean Quinoa Salad	91
162)	Power Bulgur Salad with Herbs	91
163)	ORIGINAL ROASTED Pepper Salad	92
164)	Winter Hearty Quinoa Soup	92
165)	Green Lentil Salad	93
166)	Chickpea, Acorn Squash, and Couscous Soup	93
167)	Garlic Crostini with Cabbage Soup	94

168) Green Bean Soup Cream 94
169) French Traditional Onion Soup 95
170) Roasted Carrot Soup 95
171) Italian Penne Pasta Salad 96
172) Chana Chaat Indian Salad 96
173) Tempeh and Noodle Salad Thai-Style 97
174) Typical Cream of Broccoli Soup 97
175) Raisin Moroccan Lentil Salad 98
176) Chickpea and Asparagus Salad 98
177) Quinoa and Avocado Salad 99
178) Tabbouleh Salad with Tofu 99
179) Green Pasta Salad 100
180) Original Ukrainian Borscht 101
181) Lentil Beluga Salad 101
182) Indian Naan Salad 102
183) Broccoli Ginger Soup 102
184) Noodle Rice Soup with Beans 102
185) Vegetable and Rice Soup 103
186) Daikon and Sweet Potato Soup 103
187) Chickpea and Vegetable Soup 103
188) Italian-style Bean Soup 105
189) Brussels Sprouts and Tofu Soup 105
190) White Bean Rosemary Soup 105
191) Mushroom and Tofu Soup 106
192) Autumn Root Vegetable Soup 106
193) Greek Salad 106

VEGETABLES AND SIDE DISHES 108

194) Chinese Cabbage Stir-Fry 109

195) Sautéed Cauliflower with Sesame Seeds 109

196) Sweet Mashed Carrots 110

197) Sautéed Turnip Greens 110

198) Yukon Gold Mashed Potatoes 111

199) Aromatic Sautéed Swiss Chard 111

200) Classic Sautéed Bell Peppers 111

201) Mashed Root Vegetables 112

202) Roasted Butternut Squash 112

203) Sautéed Cremini Mushrooms 112

204) Roasted Asparagus with Sesame Seeds 113

205) Greek-Style Eggplant Skillet 113

206) Cauliflower Rice 114

207) Garlicky Kale 114

208) Artichokes Braised in Lemon and Olive Oil 115

209) Rosemary and Garlic Roasted Carrots 115

LUNCH 116

210) Millet Porridge with Sultanas 117

211) Quinoa Porridge with Dried Figs 117

212) Bread Pudding with Raisins 117

213) Bulgur Wheat Salad 118

214) Rye Porridge with Blueberry Topping 118

215) Coconut Sorghum Porridge 118

216) Mum's Aromatic Rice 119

217) Everyday Savory Grits 119

218)	Greek-Style Barley Salad	119
219)	Sweet Maize Meal Porridge	120
220)	Dad's Millet Muffins	120
221)	Ginger Brown Rice	120
222)	Chili Bean and Brown Rice Tortillas	121
223)	Cashew Buttered Quesadillas with Leafy Greens	122
224)	Asparagus with Creamy Puree	122
225)	Kale Mushroom Galette	123
226)	Focaccia with Mixed Mushrooms	124
227)	Seitan Cakes with Broccoli Mash	124
228)	Spicy Cheese with Tofu Balls	125
229)	Quinoa and Veggie Burgers	125
230)	Baked Tofu with Roasted Peppers	126
231)	Zoodle Bolognese	126
232)	Zucchini Boats with Vegan Cheese	127
233)	Roasted Butternut Squash with Chimichurri	127
234)	Sweet and Spicy Brussel Sprout Stir-Fry	128
235)	Black Bean Burgers with BBQ Sauce	128
236)	Creamy Brussels Sprouts Bake	129
237)	Basil Pesto Seitan Panini	129
238)	Sweet Oatmeal "Grits"	130
239)	Freekeh Bowl with Dried Figs	130
240)	Cornmeal Porridge with Maple Syrup	130

DINNER 131

241)	Matcha-Infused Tofu Rice	132
242)	Chinese Fried Rice	132

243)	Savory Seitan xand Bell Pepper Rice	133
244)	Asparagus and Mushrooms with Mashed Potatoes	133
245)	Green Pea and Lemon Couscous	133
246)	Chimichurri Fusili with Navy Beans	134
247)	Quinoa and Chickpea Pot	134
248)	Buckwheat Pilaf with Pine Nuts	135
249)		135
250)	Italian Holiday Stuffing	135
251)	Pressure Cooker Green Lentils	135
252)	Cherry and Pistachio Bulgur	136
253)	Mushroom Fried Rice	136
254)	Bean and Brown Rice with Artichokes	136
255)	Pressure Cooker Celery and Spinach Chickpeas	137
256)	Veggie Paella with Lentils	137
257)	Curry Bean with Artichokes	138
258)	Endive Slaw with Olives	138
259)	Paprika Cauliflower Tacos	138

SNACKS 139

260)	Freekeh Salad with Za'atar	140
261)	Vegetable Amaranth Soup	140
262)	Polenta with Mushrooms and Chickpeas	141
263)	Teff Salad with Avocado and Beans	141
264)	Overnight Oatmeal with Walnuts	142
265)	Colorful Spelt Salad	142
266)	Powerful Teff Bowl with Tahini Sauce	143
267)	Polenta Toasts with Balsamic Onions	143

268)	Freekeh Pilaf with Chickpeas	144
269)	Grandma's Pilau with Garden Vegetables	144
270)	Easy Barley Risotto	145
271)	Traditional Portuguese Papas	145
272)	The Best Millet Patties Ever	145

DESSERTS 146

273)	Avocado Truffles with Chocolate Coating	147
274)	Vanilla Berry Tarts	147
275)	Homemade Chocolates with Coconut and Raisins	148
276)	Mocha Fudge	148
277)	Almond and Chocolate Chip Bars	148
278)	Almond Butter Cookies	149
279)	Peanut Butter Oatmeal Bars	149
280)	Vanilla Halvah Fudge	150
281)	Raw Chocolate Mango Pie	150
282)	Chocolate N'ice Cream	150
283)	Raw Raspberry Cheesecake	151
284)	Mini Lemon Tarts	151
285)	Coconut Blondies with Raisins	152
286)	Chocolate Squares	152
287)	Chocolate and Raisin Cookie Bars	153
288)	Almond Granola Bars	153

AUTHOR BIOGRAPHY 154

CONCLUSIONS 156

© Copyright 2021 - All rights reserved.

The content contained within this book may not be reproduced, duplicated or transmitted without direct written permission from the author or the publisher.

Under no circumstances will any blame or legal responsibility be held against the publisher, or author, for any damages, reparation, or monetary loss due to the information contained within this book, either directly or indirectly.

Legal Notice:

This book is copyright protected. It is only for personal use. You cannot amend, distribute, sell, use, quote or paraphrase any part, or the content within this book, without the consent of the author or publisher.

Disclaimer Notice:

Please note the information contained within this document is for educational and entertainment purposes only. All effort has been executed to present accurate, up to date, reliable, complete information. No warranties of any kind are declared or implied. Readers acknowledge that the author is not engaged in the rendering of legal, financial, medical or professional advice. The content within this book has been de-rived from various sources. Please consult a licensed professional before attempting any techniques out-lined in this book.

By reading this document, the reader agrees that under no circumstances is the author responsible for any losses, direct or indirect, that are incurred as a result of the use of the information contained within this document, including, but not limited to, errors, omissions, or inaccuracies.

PART 1-INTRODUCTION TO THE PLANT-BASED DIET

Vegan athletes need to be aware of what they eat and how much they eat to absorb the necessary nutrition that supports muscle function, repair, endurance, strength, and motivation. These are qualities that professional athlete's treasure. Protein is at the top of the list of things to eat. You should also consider your caloric intake, macro and micro nutritional sources, and amino acids, some of which may need to be supplemented. Protein and carbohydrates average four calories per gram, while fat averages nine calories per gram. Following this, you can calculate how much of each type of nutrient to consume per day.

When planning a vegan diet, an athlete may need to consider their exercise routines, as those who work out may have high-impact days (like the dreaded "leg-day") and low-impact days where their body needs more nutrients geared toward repair work. Their eating plan will be based solely on their age, weight, activity level, food availability (vegetables and fruits tend to be seasonal), and personal taste for each athlete. It is certainly not necessary to eat buckets of beans to be vegan.

Converting to a vegetarian diet from an omnivorous diet can, surprisingly, be a vast mental shock; however, there are also some changes to your digestive system to consider. Vegans consume more dietary fiber than most omnivores, so your intestines may go through phases where you feel a bit bloated. You will need to consume more water. There are many suggested ratios, but the simplest is to work on a per calorie basis. A quick rule of 1 milliliter of water per calorie seems easy enough to follow. Keeping in mind that your food volume may increase, you may also need to eat a little earlier than an omnivore would before exercising. So, the usual rule of one hour of fasting before eating may need to be extended to 90 minutes of fasting before exercising.

Always consider adding variety to your vegan diet, as this increases your body's ability to consume all the vital amino acids, leading to better protein synthesis (which is essential for developing muscle tone and recovering from injuries). Plant-based meals are very satiating due to their high fiber content, but you need to consume more of them to meet your calorie needs. To avoid feeling too full, you can get extra carbs by eating nuts and seeds throughout the day as snacks.

Finally, when adding the finishing touches to your workout program, it's essential to intersperse your training sessions with enough time to ensure your muscles have time to rest and recover (where you rebuild your energy reserves, hydrate your body, and restore your metabolism's normal chemical balance). Short-term rest periods can be anything from taking a break for a few minutes before moving on to the next training activity or even taking the rest of the day off after a particularly strenuous session. Professional athletes know that the body may be a machine, but it's a machine that needs to have "downtime" as well. It would be best to make a training journal in which you record what you ate, how long you fasted before your workout, and how you felt during and after your training session. This will help you assess whether you need to add more carbs or protein to your diet and whether you need a longer rest period before moving on to the next training activity.

If you struggle with fatigue (or shakes) after strenuous activities, you may need to increase your amino acid intake or get more zinc and iron into your system. We are all unique, and what works for another vegan athlete may not work for you. This training log can also allow you to experiment by perhaps switching to shorter training sessions with more frequent rest periods to achieve the same fitness and muscle-building level. No two professional athletes train the same way. Listen to your body and your instincts to find a way that works for you.

Finally, don't forget to get enough sleep. Mental fatigue can easily translate into physical symptoms. A magnesium deficiency can also cause insomnia. This could be caused by strenuous activity that uses up the body's natural minerals. Taking a magnesium supplement or eating some dark chocolate or half a banana before bed can help create restful sleep.

Fortunately, the Internet allows for the development of support networks for vegan athletes. What we eat says a lot about us, and vegans can be successful, high-level athletes with planning and experimentation to find what works for their unique bodies.

THE BENEFITS OF THE PLANT-BASED DIET

A plant-based diet has proven health effects due to its food composition. Reduced saturated fat consumption prevents various diseases, including cardiovascular problems, high cholesterol levels, and obesity. The following are other guaranteed benefits of this diet:

WEIGHT AND BMI CONTROL

Research studies conducted on the plant-based diet have revealed that people who follow it tend to have a lower BMI or body mass index, reduced risk of obesity, and a lower likelihood of heart disease and diabetes. This is mainly because plant-based diets provide more fiber, water, and carbohydrates to the body. This can keep the body's metabolism active and functioning properly while providing a good boost of continuous energy.

In 2018, a study was conducted on this diet plan, and it was found to be the most effective in treating obesity. In that study, 75 people with obesity or weight issues were given a completely vegan plant-based diet, and their results were compared to those consuming animal-based diets. After four months of this experiment, the plant-based diet group showed a significant decrease in their body weight (up to 6.5 kilograms). Everyone lost more fat mass and demonstrated improved insulin sensitivity. Another study involving 60,000 individuals showed similar results, with people following a vegan diet recording lower body mass index than vegetarians and those following a plant-based diet.

Lower risk of heart disease and other conditions

The American Heart Association recently conducted a study in which middle-aged adults who followed a plant-based diet were studied. All of the subjects showed a decrease in their rate of heart disease. Based on the results of this research, the association listed the following illnesses that can be prevented through a plant-based diet:

- Heart attack
- High blood pressure
- High cholesterol levels
- Certain types of cancer
- Type II diabetes
- Obesity
- Diabetes

Plant-based diets also help manage diabetes because they improve insulin sensitivity and combat insulin resistance. Of all 60,000 study participants, about 2.9% on the vegan diet had type II diabetes, while 7.6% of participants on non-vegetarian diets had type II diabetes. From this observation, the researchers confirmed that a plant-based diet could help in the treatment of diabetes. It has also been proposed that this diet may help diabetic patients lose weight, improve metabolic rate and decrease their need for medical treatment.

It has also been suggested that doctors recommend this diet as part of treating people with type II diabetes or prediabetes. While medical treatments ensure short-term results, the plant-based dietary approach offers long-term results.

HOW TO START TO LOSE WEIGHT

Collect recipes for the meals you will be making.
Organize your list. You can divide the meals into groups, for example, soups, meat dishes, vegetarian dishes and so on, so that it is easy to manage them.
Find the recipes you need and write them down or print them on sheets of paper. Also, you can consider buying a special notebook for recipes. The most important thing is to have easy access to them because you will need them often.

Write your menu on paper
You have many ways to do this. You can use a notebook. On the other side, write a list of your meals, and on the right side, write down all the ingredients needed to prepare this meal (at once, you will have a meal plan and shopping list).
Regardless of which method you choose, put your plan in a visible place for everyone in the house. The best site is in the kitchen.

Adapt the menu according to your family's eventualities
When planning your meals, consider your daily activities and those of your family. Did your children eat lunch at school? Plan a more modest lunch at home that day. Are you coming home late from work? Think about a dinner that takes little time to prepare. Has the family been invited to a Sunday dinner? You don't have to prepare dinner that day. It is good to consider all related factors and take them into account when creating the menu.

Make a list of 15-20 of your favorite foods.
To make this list, sit down with your whole family and ask everyone what their favorite foods are. Once you've done that, look at the list and select those quick and easy to prepare and don't need too many ingredients. Best if they are healthy meals.

Check what you have in your pantry
Before you put your menu in place, it's a good idea to check your pantry, refrigerator, and freezer. Organize all the food you have there: throw away what is already expired, and sort everything else into appropriate groups (go to the shopping list template to see an example of groups)
Plan meals based on the products you already have. For example, do you have pasta? Put the pasta on your grocery list for the next day. If you like chicken pasta but don't have it, write "chicken" on your grocery list.
This way, you'll cut down on your grocery bill and also avoid unnecessary purchases of products you already have at home. Plus, it's the first step to keeping your refrigerator and pantry in order.

Use seasonal products

Depending on the season, the availability of individual fruits and vegetables can change drastically. As a result, their prices change as well. The best prices are found during the harvest, which becomes saving. The bottom line is that it's normal for your menu to change throughout the year.
I recommend using fresh ingredients from your garden season or those available in the market this season.

Plan meals throughout the day

Don't just create a list of lunches. It is advisable to eat 3-5 times a day, so think about planning all your breakfasts, lunches, and dinners.
This will prevent you from eating out, help you plan and make better use of your cooking time. You will also have the opportunity to use better leftover food (this is important if you want to maximize the savings effect).

Plan your food clean-up day

If you ever collect all the leftovers from your refrigerator at the end of the week, you can plan an evening when you and your family will dine on only the leftovers.
On that day, you should also check which products are close to the expiration date, and these are the products to be used in the following days' meals. This will reduce food waste and save you money.

Prepare multiple meals at once

Are you planning to eat the same dish more than once during the week? Try preparing a more significant amount of this meal for today and the next few days. If you do, put the food separately in containers and put them in the refrigerator or freezer; you can also bottle the food in jars.
Another example: you make chicken breast chops for lunch, and you also like a salad with chicken breast. Cook more than a single chicken breast at a time and then store some in the refrigerator. As a result, you will prepare the salad much faster in the afternoon or the next day.

Review your daily plan

Your meal plan should be flexible. If necessary, don't be afraid to make adjustments and take advantage of opportunities.
Many people consider themselves picky about food before they switch to a plant-based diet. However, then you find foods that they couldn't even think. Beans, tofu, different kinds of sweets from plants - such a meal for a meat lover seems tasteless. So, try a new dish and let your taste buds decide for themselves what they like best.

The Plant-Based for Athlete

THE FUNDAMENTAL FACTORS FOR BEING FIT

It is not easy to make a change in any diet that you quickly embrace. The decision to embark on a plant-based eating plan is based on a desire to live a healthier life. Change may be inevitable later, after many realizations of what we get when we eventually abandon what we prefer to consume.

1. The first tip is about creating a consistent trend towards plant-based meals. Make a plan to cook this food more often within a week. Don't wait until ages have passed since you are inducing yourself to start your plant-based diet. Practice makes perfect, and within a long time, your skills, especially the necessary ones, will improve. Your experience will be a notch higher, and this will be reflected in your habits. Making it a point to cook plant-based meals frequently is one of the most excellent tips to start your plant-based meal. Along the way, you will adapt to it. You'll also find that you've changed your approach from how you've always thought about other types of food, such as diets filled with meat and junk food.

2. One tip that will help you start a plant-based diet meal is the use of whole grains during breakfast. Use them in large quantities, as they will help you to adopt this type of diet in a short period. It is not always easy to use all these whole grains. The best way to go about it is to choose meals that can satisfy you and the rest of your family at first. Good examples will be highly recommended. These could include oats, barley, or even buckwheat. Here, you can add some flavors provided by different types of nuts and other seeds. Don't forget to include fresh fruit alongside your entree.

3. The next tip is about making rules and making sure you are initiated into new plant-based meal recipes even twice a week. Regulations created by yourself will be followed quickly than those formed and forced on you. In this plant-based diet, it is all about loving what you are doing. The recipes you create will always be easy to follow, and once you master them, you will only get better at them. One rule that can be created here is the setting of a day. This day is kept mainly for one purpose, and that is to make a plant-based meal. Do this to the family and get their final verdict on what you did. Ask them to comment on the tastes and the food in general. The result will help you a lot, especially in your next meal.

4. Another tip is about food pairing. You can use this tool to have a more excellent knowledge of what types of plant-based foods can be paired and good taste results. You can do this pairing by combining different flavors. The result should give you a strong feeling that works for you.

5. As a beginner in this diet, the best tip for starting a plant-based eating plan will be, to begin with, vegetables. Try your best to eat vegetables. The act can be during lunch and dinner or rather a dinner. Make sure that your plate is always filled with plants from different categories. The different colors can help you choose the different types that you want to learn. Vegetables can also be eaten as snacks, especially when combined with hummus or salsa. You can also use guacamole in this combination, and rest assured you will love it.

The Plant-Based for Athlete

Breakfast

BREAKFAST

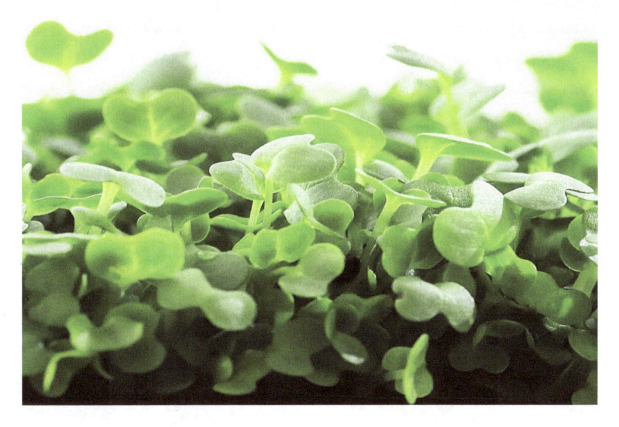

The Plant-Based for Athlete

1) KID-FRIENDLY CEREAL

Preparation Time: 15 minutes

Servings: 5

Ingredients:

- 1 ½ cups spelt flour
- 1/2 tsp baking powder
- 1 tsp cinnamon
- 1/2 tsp cardamom
- 1/4 tsp ground cloves
- 1/2 cup brown sugar
- 1/3 cup almond milk
- 2 tsp coconut oil, melted

Directions:

- Begin by preheating your oven to 350 degrees F.
- In a mixing bowl, thoroughly combine all the dry ingredients. Gradually, pour in the milk and coconut oil and mix to combine well.
- Fill the pastry bag with the batter. Now, pipe 1/4-inch balls onto parchment-lined cookie sheets.
- Bake in the preheated oven for about 13 minutes. Serve with your favorite plant-based milk.
- Store in an air-thigh container for about 1 month. Enjoy

2) ORIGINAL BREAKFAST BURRITO

Preparation Time: 15 minutes

Servings: 4

Ingredients:

- 1 tbsp olive oil
- 16 ounces tofu, pressed
- 4 (6-inch) whole-wheat tortillas
- 1 ½ cups canned chickpeas, drained
- 1 medium-sized avocado, pitted and sliced
- 1 tbsp lemon juice
- 1 tsp garlic, pressed
- 2 bell peppers, sliced
- Sea salt and ground black pepper, to taste
- 1/2 tsp red pepper flakes

Directions:

- Heat the olive oil in a frying skillet over medium heat. When it's hot, add the tofu and sauté for about 10 minutes, stirring occasionally to promote even cooking.
- Divide the fried tofu between warmed tortillas; place the remaining ingredients on your tortillas, roll them up and serve immediately.
- Enjoy

3) HOMEMADE TOAST CRUNCH

Preparation Time: 15 minutes

Servings: 8

Ingredients:

- 1 cup almond flour
- 1 cup coconut flour
- 1/2 cup all-purpose flour
- 1 cup sugar
- 1 tsp kosher salt
- 1 tsp cardamom
- 1/4 tsp grated nutmeg
- 1 tbsp cinnamon
- 3 tbsp flax seeds, ground
- 1/2 cup coconut oil, melted
- 8 tbsp coconut milk

Directions:

- Begin by preheating the oven to 340 degrees F. In a mixing bowl, thoroughly combine all the dry ingredients.
- Gradually pour in the oil and milk; mix to combine well.
- Shape the dough into a ball and roll out between 2 sheets of a parchment paper. Cut into small squares and prick them with a fork to prevent air bubbles.
- Bake in the preheated oven for about 15 minutes. They will continue to crisp as they cool. Enjoy!

4) CINNAMON AND APPLE OATMEAL CUPS

Preparation Time: 30 minutes

Servings: 9

Ingredients:

- 2 cups old-fashioned oats
- 1/2 tsp baking powder
- 1 tsp cinnamon
- 1/4 tsp grated nutmeg
- 1/4 tsp sea salt
- 1 cup almond milk
- 1/4 cup agave syrup
- 1/2 cup applesauce
- 2 tbsp coconut oil
- 2 tbsp peanut butter
- 1 tbsp chia seeds
- 1 small apple, cored and diced

Directions:

- Begin by preheating your oven to 360 degrees F. Spritz a muffin tin with a nonstick cooking oil.
- In a mixing bowl, thoroughly combine all the ingredients, except for the apples.
- Fold in the apples and scrape the batter into the prepared muffin tin.
- Bake your muffins for about 25 minutes or until a toothpick comes out dry and clean. Enjoy

5) CHICKPEA TOFU SCRAMBLE WITH SPICY VEGETABLES

Preparation Time: 15 minutes

Servings: 2

Ingredients:

- 2 tbsp oil
- 1 bell pepper, seeded and sliced
- 2 tbsp scallions, chopped
- 6 ounces cremini button mushrooms, sliced
- 1/2 tsp garlic, minced
- 1 jalapeno pepper, seeded and chopped
- 6 ounces firm tofu, pressed
- 1 tbsp nutritional yeast
- 1/4 tsp turmeric powder
- Kala namak and ground black pepper, to taste
- 6 ounces chickpeas, drained

Directions:

- Heat the olive oil in a nonstick skillet over a moderate flame. Once hot, sauté the pepper for about 2 minutes.
- Now, add in the scallions, mushrooms and continue sautéing for a further 3 minutes or until the mushrooms release the liquid.
- Then, add in the garlic, jalapeno and tofu and sauté for 5 minutes more, crumbling the tofu with a fork.
- Add in the nutritional yeast, turmeric, salt, pepper and chickpeas; continue sautéing an additional 2 minutes or until cooked through. Enjoy

6) COCONUT PRUNES GRANOLA

Preparation Time: 1 hour

Servings: 10

Ingredients:

- 1/3 cup coconut oil
- 1/2 cup maple syrup
- 1 tsp sea salt
- 1/4 tsp grated nutmeg
- 1/2 tsp cinnamon powder
- 1/2 tsp vanilla extract
- 4 cups old-fashioned oats
- 1/2 cup almonds, chopped
- 1/2 cup pecans, chopped
- 1/2 coconut, shredded
- 1 cup prunes, chopped

Directions:

- Begin by preheating your oven to 260 degrees F; line two rimmed baking sheets with a piece of parchment paper.
- Then, thoroughly combine the coconut oil, maple syrup, salt, nutmeg, cinnamon and vanilla.
- Gradually add in the oats, almonds, pecans and coconut; toss to coat well.
- Spread the mixture out onto the prepared baking sheets.
- Bake in the middle of the oven, stirring halfway through the cooking time, for about 1 hour or until golden brown.
- Stir in the prunes and let your granola cool completely before storing. Store in an airtight container.
- Enjoy

7) THYME PUMPKIN FRY

Preparation Time: 25 minutes

Servings: 2

Ingredients:

- 1 cup pumpkin, shredded
- 1 tbsp olive oil
- ½ onion, chopped
- 1 carrot, peeled and chopped
- 2 garlic cloves, minced
- ½ tsp dried thyme
- 1 cup chopped kale
- Salt and black pepper to taste

Directions:

- Heat the oil in a skillet over medium heat. Sauté onion and carrot for 5 minutes. Add in garlic and thyme, cook for 30 seconds until the garlic is fragrant. Place in the pumpkin and cook for 10 minutes until tender. Stir in kale, cook for 4 minutes until the kale wilts. Season with salt and pepper. Serve hot

8) ALMOND RASPBERRY SMOOTHIE

Preparation Time: 5 minutes

Servings: 4

Ingredients:

- 1 ½ cups almond milk
- ½ cup raspberries
- Juice from half lemon
- ½ tsp almond extract

Directions:

- In a blender or smoothie maker, pour the almond milk, raspberries, lemon juice, and almond extract. Puree the ingredients at high speed until the raspberries have blended almost entirely into the liquid. Pour the smoothie into serving glasses. Stick in some straws and serve immediately

9) KIWI OATMEAL BARS

Preparation Time: 50 minutes

Servings: 12

Ingredients:

- 2 cups uncooked rolled oats
- 2 cups all-purpose flour
- 1 ½ cups pure date sugar
- 1 ½ tsp baking soda
- ½ tsp ground cinnamon
- 1 cup plant butter, melted
- 4 cups kiwi, chopped
- ¼ cup organic cane sugar
- 2 tbsp corn-starch

Directions:

- Preheat oven to 380 F. Grease a baking dish.
- In a bowl, mix the oats, flour, date sugar, baking soda, salt, and cinnamon. Put in butter and whisk to combine. In another bowl, combine the kiwis, cane sugar, and corn-starch until the kiwis are coated. Spread 3 cups of oatmeal mixture on a greased baking dish and top with kiwi mixture and finally put the remaining oatmeal mixture on top. Bake for 40 minutes. Allow cooling and slice into bars

10) APPLE SPICY PANCAKES

Preparation Time: 30 minutes

Servings: 4

Ingredients:

- 2 cups almond milk
- 1 tsp apple cider vinegar
- 2 ½ cups whole-wheat flour
- 2 tbsp baking powder
- ½ tsp baking soda
- 1 tsp sea salt
- ½ tsp ground cinnamon
- ¼ tsp grated nutmeg
- ¼ tsp ground allspice
- ½ cup applesauce
- 1 cup water
- 1 tbsp coconut oil

Directions:

- Whisk the almond milk and apple cider vinegar in a bowl and set aside. In another bowl, combine the flour, baking powder, baking soda, salt, cinnamon, nutmeg, and allspice. Transfer the almond mixture to another bowl and beat with the applesauce and water.
- Pour in the dry ingredients and stir. Melt some coconut oil in a skillet over medium heat. Pour a ladle of the batter and cook for 5 minutes, flipping once until golden. Repeat the process until the batter is exhausted. Serve

11) ALMOND AND COCONUT GRANOLA WITH CHERRIES

Preparation Time: 45 minutes

Servings: 6

Ingredients:

- ½ cup coconut oil, melted
- ½ cup maple syrup
- 1 tsp vanilla extract
- 3 tsp pumpkin pie spice
- 4 cups rolled oats
- ⅓ cup whole-wheat flour
- ¼ cup ground flaxseed
- ½ cup sunflower seeds
- ½ cup slivered almonds
- ½ cup shredded coconut
- ½ cup dried cherries
- ½ cup dried apricots, chopped

Directions:

- Preheat oven to 350 F.
- In a bowl, combine the coconut oil, maple syrup, and vanilla. Add in the pumpkin pie spice. Put oats, flour, flaxseed, sunflower seeds, almonds, and coconut in a baking sheet and toss to combine. Coat with the oil mixture. Spread the granola out evenly. Bake for 25 minutes. Once ready, break the granola into chunks and stir in the cherries and apricots. Bake another 5 minutes. Allow cooling and serve

12) ALMONDS CINNAMON BUCKWHEAT

Preparation Time: 20 minutes

Servings: 4

Ingredients:

- 1 cup almond milk
- 1 cup water
- 1 cup buckwheat groats, rinsed
- 1 tsp cinnamon
- ¼ cup chopped almonds
- 2 tbsp pure date syrup

Directions:

- Place almond milk, water, and buckwheat in a pot over medium heat and bring to a boil. Lower the heat and simmer covered for 15 minutes. Allow sitting covered for 5 minutes. Mix in the cinnamon, almonds, and date syrup. Serve warm

13) YELLOW SMOOTHIE

Preparation Time: 5 minutes

Servings: 4

Ingredients:
- 1 banana
- 1 cup chopped mango
- 1 cup chopped apricots
- 1 cup strawberries
- 1 carrot, peeled and chopped
- 1 cup water

Directions:
- Put the banana, mango, apricots, strawberries, carrot, and water in a food processor. Pulse until smooth; add more water if needed. Divide between glasses and serve

14) HEARTY SMOOTHIE

Preparation Time: 5 minutes

Servings: 3

Ingredients:
- 1 banana
- ½ cup coconut milk
- 1 cup water
- 1 cup broccoli sprouts
- 2 cherries, pitted
- 1 tbsp hemp hearts
- ¼ tsp ground cinnamon
- ¼ tsp ground cardamom
- 1 tbsp grated fresh ginger

Directions:
- In a food processor, place banana, coconut milk, water, broccoli, cherries, hemp hearts, cinnamon, cardamom, and ginger. Blitz until smooth. Divide between glasses and serve

15) CARROT AND STRAWBERRY SMOOTHIE

Preparation Time: 5 minutes

Servings: 2

Ingredients:
- 1 cup peeled and diced carrots
- 1 cup strawberries
- 1 apple, chopped
- 2 tbsp maple syrup
- 2 cups unsweetened almond milk

Directions:
- Place in a food processor all the ingredients. Blitz until smooth. Pour in glasses and serve

16) SUPER GREEN SMOOTHIE

Preparation Time: 10 minutes

Servings: 2

Ingredients:
- 1 banana, sliced
- 2 cups kale
- 1 cup sliced kiwi
- 1 orange, cut into segments
- 1 cup unsweetened coconut milk

Directions:
- In a food processor, put the banana, kale, kiwi, orange, and coconut milk. Pulse until smooth. Serve right away in glasses

17) BLUEBERRY MAPLE SMOOTHIE

Preparation Time: 5 minutes

Servings: 4

Ingredients:
- 4 cups chopped arugula
- 2 cups frozen blueberries
- 4 cups unsweetened almond milk
- Juice of 2 limes
- 4 tbsp maple syrup

Directions:
- In a food processor, blitz the arugula, blueberries, almond milk, lime juice, and maple syrup until smooth. Serve

18) POWER CHIA-PEACH SMOOTHIE

Preparation Time: 5 minutes

Servings: 2

Ingredients:

- 1 banana, sliced
- 1 peach, chopped
- 1 cup almond milk
- 1 scoop plant-based protein powder
- 1 tbsp chia seeds
- 1 cucumber, chopped

Directions:

- Purée the banana, peach, almond milk, protein powder, chia seeds, and cucumber for 50 seconds until smooth in a food processor. Serve immediately in glasses

19) PORRIDGE WITH STRAWBERRIES AND COCONUT

Preparation Time: 12 minutes

Servings: 2

Ingredients:

- 1 tbsp flax seed powder
- 1 oz olive oil
- 1 tbsp coconut flour
- 1 pinch ground chia seeds
- 5 tbsp coconut cream
- Thawed frozen strawberries

Directions:

- In a small bowl, mix the flax seed powder with the 3 tbsp water, and allow soaking for 5 minutes.
- Place a non-stick saucepan over low heat and pour in the olive oil, vegan "flax egg," coconut flour, chia seeds, and coconut cream.
- Cook the mixture while stirring continuously until your desired consistency is achieved. Turn the heat off and spoon the porridge into serving bowls.
- Top with 4 to 6 strawberries and serve immediately.

20) BROCCOLI BROWNS

Preparation Time: 35 minutes

Servings: 4

Ingredients:

- 3 tbsp flax seed powder
- 1 head broccoli, cut into florets
- ½ white onion, grated
- 1 tsp salt
- 1 tbsp freshly ground black pepper
- 5 tbsp plant butter, for frying

Directions:

- In a small bowl, mix the flax seed powder with 9 tbsp water, and allow soaking for 5 minutes. Pour the broccoli into a food processor and pulse a few times until smoothly grated.
- Transfer the broccoli into a bowl, add the vegan "flax egg," white onion, salt, and black pepper. Use a spoon to mix the ingredients evenly and set aside 5 to 10 minutes to firm up a bit. Place a large non-stick skillet over medium heat and drop 1/3 of the plant butter to melt until no longer shimmering.
- Ladle scoops of the broccoli mixture into the skillet (about 3 to 4 hash browns per batch). Flatten the pancakes to measure 3 to 4 inches in diameter, and fry until golden brown on one side, 4 minutes. Turn the pancakes with a spatula and cook the other side to brown too, another 5 minutes.
- Transfer the hash browns to a serving plate and repeat the frying process for the remaining broccoli mixture. Serve the hash browns warm with green salad.

The Plant-Based for Athlete

Soups, Stew, and Salads

SOUPS, STEW AND SALADS

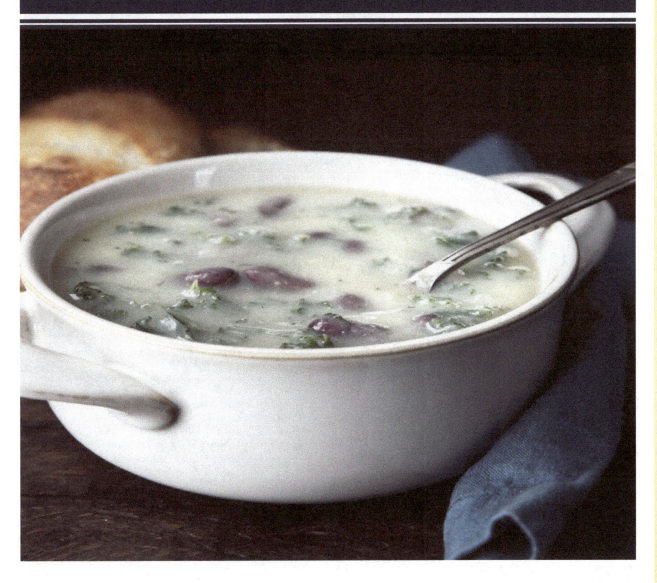

21) ROASTED CARROT SOUP

Preparation Time: 50 minutes

Servings: 4

Ingredients:

- 1 ½ pounds carrots
- 4 tbsp olive oil
- 1 yellow onion, chopped
- 2 cloves garlic, minced
- 1/3 tsp ground cumin
- Sea salt and white pepper, to taste
- 1/2 tsp turmeric powder
- 4 cups vegetable stock
- 2 tsp lemon juice
- 2 tbsp fresh cilantro, roughly chopped

Directions:

- Start by preheating your oven to 400 degrees F. Place the carrots on a large parchment-lined baking sheet; toss the carrots with 2 tbsp of the olive oil.
- Roast the carrots for about 35 minutes or until they've softened.
- In a heavy-bottomed pot, heat the remaining 2 tbsp of the olive oil. Now, sauté the onion and garlic for about 3 minutes or until aromatic.
- Add in the cumin, salt, pepper, turmeric, vegetable stock and roasted carrots. Continue to simmer for 12 minutes more.
- Puree your soup with an immersion blender. Drizzle lemon juice over your soup and serve garnished with fresh cilantro leaves. Enjoy

22) ITALIAN PENNE PASTA SALAD

Preparation Time: 15 minutes + chilling time

Servings: 3

Ingredients:

- 9 ounces penne pasta
- 9 ounces canned Cannellini bean, drained
- 1 small onion, thinly sliced
- 1/3 cup Niçoise olives, pitted and sliced
- 2 Italian peppers, sliced
- 1 cup cherry tomatoes, halved
- 3 cups arugula
- Dressing:
- 3 tbsp extra-virgin olive oil
- 1 tsp lemon zest
- 1 tsp garlic, minced
- 3 tbsp balsamic vinegar
- 1 tsp Italian herb mix
- Sea salt and ground black pepper, to taste

Directions:

- Cook the penne pasta according to the package directions. Drain and rinse the pasta. Let it cool completely and then, transfer it to a salad bowl.
- Then, add the beans, onion, olives, peppers, tomatoes and arugula to the salad bowl.
- Mix all the dressing ingredients until everything is well incorporated. Dress your salad and serve well

23) CHANA CHAAT INDIAN SALAD

Preparation Time: 45 minutes + chilling time

Servings: 4

Ingredients:

- 1 pound dry chickpeas, soaked overnight
- 2 San Marzano tomatoes, diced
- 1 Persian cucumber, sliced
- 1 onion, chopped
- 1 bell pepper, seeded and thinly sliced
- 1 green chili, seeded and thinly sliced
- 2 handfuls baby spinach
- 1/2 tsp Kashmiri chili powder
- 4 curry leaves, chopped
- 1 tbsp chaat masala
- 2 tbsp fresh lemon juice, or to taste
- 4 tbsp olive oil
- 1 tsp agave syrup
- 1/2 tsp mustard seeds
- 1/2 tsp coriander seeds
- 2 tbsp sesame seeds, lightly toasted
- 2 tbsp fresh cilantro, roughly chopped

Directions:

- Drain the chickpeas and transfer them to a large saucepan. Cover the chickpeas with water by 2 inches and bring it to a boil.
- Immediately turn the heat to a simmer and continue to cook for approximately 40 minutes.
- Toss the chickpeas with the tomatoes, cucumber, onion, peppers, spinach, chili powder, curry leaves and chaat masala.
- In a small mixing dish, thoroughly combine the lemon juice, olive oil, agave syrup, mustard seeds and coriander seeds.
- Garnish with sesame seeds and fresh cilantro. Enjoy

24) TEMPEH AND NOODLE SALAD THAI-STYLE

Preparation Time: 45 minutes

Servings: 3

Ingredients:

- 6 ounces tempeh
- 4 tbsp rice vinegar
- 4 tbsp soy sauce
- 2 garlic cloves, minced
- 1 small-sized lime, freshly juiced
- 5 ounces rice noodles
- 1 carrot, julienned
- 1 shallot, chopped
- 3 handfuls Chinese cabbage, thinly sliced
- 3 handfuls kale, torn into pieces
- 1 bell pepper, seeded and thinly sliced
- 1 bird's eye chili, minced
- 1/4 cup peanut butter
- 2 tbsp agave syrup

Directions:

- Place the tempeh, 2 tbsp of the rice vinegar, soy sauce, garlic and lime juice in a ceramic dish; let it marinate for about 40 minutes.
- Meanwhile, cook the rice noodles according to the package directions. Drain your noodles and transfer them to a salad bowl.
- Add the carrot, shallot, cabbage, kale and peppers to the salad bowl. Add in the peanut butter, the remaining 2 tbsp of the rice vinegar and agave syrup and toss to combine well.
- Top with the marinated tempeh and serve immediately. Enjoy

25) TYPICAL CREAM OF BROCCOLI SOUP

Preparation Time: 35 minutes

Servings: 4

Ingredients:

- 2 tbsp olive oil
- 1 pound broccoli florets
- 1 onion, chopped
- 1 celery rib, chopped
- 1 parsnip, chopped
- 1 tsp garlic, chopped
- 3 cups vegetable broth
- 1/2 tsp dried dill
- 1/2 tsp dried oregano
- Sea salt and ground black pepper, to taste
- 2 tbsp flaxseed meal
- 1 cup full-fat coconut milk

Directions:

- In a heavy-bottomed pot, heat the olive oil over medium-high heat. Now, sauté the broccoli onion, celery and parsnip for about 5 minutes, stirring periodically.
- Add in the garlic and continue sautéing for 1 minute or until fragrant.
- Then, stir in the vegetable broth, dill, oregano, salt and black pepper; bring to a boil. Immediately reduce the heat to a simmer and let it cook for about 20 minutes.
- Puree the soup using an immersion blender until creamy and uniform.
- Return the pureed mixture to the pot. Fold in the flaxseed meal and coconut milk; continue to simmer until heated through or about 5 minutes.
- Ladle into four serving bowls and enjoy

26) RAISIN MOROCCAN LENTIL SALAD

Preparation Time: 20 minutes + chilling time

Servings: 4

Ingredients:

- 1 cup red lentils, rinsed
- 1 large carrot, julienned
- 1 Persian cucumber, thinly sliced
- 1 sweet onion, chopped
- 1/2 cup golden raisins
- 1/4 cup fresh mint, snipped
- 1/4 cup fresh basil, snipped
- 1/4 cup extra-virgin olive oil
- 1/4 cup lemon juice, freshly squeezed
- 1 tsp grated lemon peel
- 1/2 tsp fresh ginger root, peeled and minced
- 1/2 tsp granulated garlic
- 1 tsp ground allspice
- Sea salt and ground black pepper, to taste

Directions:

- In a large-sized saucepan, bring 3 cups of the water and 1 cup of the lentils to a boil.
- Immediately turn the heat to a simmer and continue to cook your lentils for a further 15 to 17 minutes or until they've softened but are not mushy yet. Drain and let it cool completely.
- Transfer the lentils to a salad bowl; add in the carrot, cucumber and sweet onion. Then, add the raisins, mint and basil to your salad.
- In a small mixing dish, whisk the olive oil, lemon juice, lemon peel, ginger, granulated garlic, allspice, salt and black pepper.
- Dress your salad and serve well-chilled. Enjoy

27) CHICKPEA AND ASPARAGUS SALAD

Preparation Time: 10 minutes + chilling time

Servings: 5

Ingredients:

- 1 ¼ pounds asparagus, trimmed and cut into bite-sized pieces
- 5 ounces canned chickpeas, drained and rinsed
- 1 chipotle pepper, seeded and chopped
- 1 Italian pepper, seeded and chopped
- 1/4 cup fresh basil leaves, chopped
- 1/4 cup fresh parsley leaves, chopped
- 2 tbsp fresh mint leaves
- 2 tbsp fresh chives, chopped
- 1 tsp garlic, minced
- 1/4 cup extra-virgin olive oil
- 1 tbsp balsamic vinegar
- 1 tbsp fresh lime juice
- 2 tbsp soy sauce
- 1/4 tsp ground allspice
- 1/4 tsp ground cumin
- Sea salt and freshly cracked peppercorns, to taste

Directions:

- Bring a large pot of salted water with the asparagus to a boil; let it cook for 2 minutes; drain and rinse.
- Transfer the asparagus to a salad bowl.
- Toss the asparagus with the chickpeas, peppers, herbs, garlic, olive oil, vinegar, lime juice, soy sauce and spices.
- Toss to combine and serve immediately. Enjoy

28) OLD-FASHIONED GREEN BEAN SALAD

Preparation Time: 10 minutes + chilling time

Servings: 4

Ingredients:

- 1 ½ pounds green beans, trimmed
- 1/2 cup scallions, chopped
- 1 tsp garlic, minced
- 1 Persian cucumber, sliced
- 2 cups grape tomatoes, halved
- 1/4 cup olive oil
- 1 tsp deli mustard
- 2 tbsp tamari sauce
- 2 tbsp lemon juice
- 1 tbsp apple cider vinegar
- 1/4 tsp cumin powder
- 1/2 tsp dried thyme
- Sea salt and ground black pepper, to taste

Directions:

- Boil the green beans in a large saucepan of salted water until they are just tender or about 2 minutes.
- Drain and let the beans cool completely; then, transfer them to a salad bowl. Toss the beans with the remaining ingredients.
- Enjoy

29) WINTER BEAN SOUP

Preparation Time: 25 minutes

Servings: 4

Ingredients:

- 1 tbsp olive oil
- 2 tbsp shallots, chopped
- 1 carrot, chopped
- 1 parsnip, chopped
- 1 celery stalk, chopped
- 1 tsp fresh garlic, minced
- 4 cups vegetable broth
- 2 bay leaves
- 1 rosemary sprig, chopped
- 16 ounces canned navy beans
- Flaky sea salt and ground black pepper, to taste

Directions:

- In a heavy-bottomed pot, heat the olive over medium-high heat. Now, sauté the shallots, carrot, parsnip and celery for approximately 3 minutes or until the vegetables are just tender.
- Add in the garlic and continue to sauté for 1 minute or until aromatic.
- Then, add in the vegetable broth, bay leaves and rosemary and bring to a boil. Immediately reduce the heat to a simmer and let it cook for 10 minutes.
- Fold in the navy beans and continue to simmer for about 5 minutes longer until everything is thoroughly heated. Season with salt and black pepper to taste.
- Ladle into individual bowls, discard the bay leaves and serve hot. Enjoy

30) ITALIAN-STYLE CREAM MUSHROOMS SOUP

Preparation Time: 15 minutes

Servings: 3

Ingredients:

- 3 tbsp vegan butter
- 1 white onion, chopped
- 1 red bell pepper, chopped
- 1/2 tsp garlic, pressed
- 3 cups Cremini mushrooms, chopped
- 2 tbsp almond flour
- 3 cups water
- 1 tsp Italian herb mix
- Sea salt and ground black pepper, to taste
- 1 heaping tbsp fresh chives, roughly chopped

Directions:

- In a stockpot, melt the vegan butter over medium-high heat. Once hot, sauté the onion and pepper for about 3 minutes until they have softened.
- Add in the garlic and Cremini mushrooms and continue sautéing until the mushrooms have softened. Sprinkle almond meal over the mushrooms and continue to cook for 1 minute or so.
- Add in the remaining ingredients. Let it simmer, covered and continue to cook for 5 to 6 minutes more until the liquid has thickened slightly.
- Ladle into three soup bowls and garnish with fresh chives. Enjoy

31) ROASTED BASIL AND TOMATO SOUP

Preparation Time: 60 minutes

Servings: 4

Ingredients:

- 2 lb tomatoes, halved
- 2 tsp garlic powder
- 3 tbsp olive oil
- 1 tbsp balsamic vinegar
- Salt and black pepper to taste
- 4 shallots, chopped
- 2 cups vegetable broth
- ½ cup basil leaves, chopped

Directions:

- Preheat oven to 450 F.
- In a bowl, mix tomatoes, garlic, 2 tbsp of oil, vinegar, salt, and pepper. Arrange the tomatoes onto a baking dish. Sprinkle with some olive oil, garlic powder, balsamic vinegar, salt, and pepper. Bake for 30 minutes until the tomatoes get dark brown color. Take out from the oven; reserve.
- Heat the remaining oil in a pot over medium heat. Place the shallots and cook for 3 minutes, stirring often. Add in roasted tomatoes and broth. Bring to a boil, then lower the heat and simmer for 10 minutes. Transfer to a food processor and blitz the soup until smooth. Serve topped with basil

32) UNDER PRESSURE COOKER GREEN ONION AND POTATO SOUP

Preparation Time: 25 minutes

Servings: 5

Ingredients:

- 3 green onions, chopped
- 4 garlic cloves, minced
- 1 tbsp olive oil
- 6 russet potatoes, chopped
- ½ (13.5-oz) can coconut milk
- 5 cups vegetable broth
- Salt and black pepper to taste

Directions:

- Set your IP to Sauté. Place in green onions, garlic, and olive oil. Cook for 3 minutes until softened. Add in potatoes, coconut milk, broth, and salt. Lock the lid in place, set time to 6 minutes on High. Once ready, perform a natural pressure release for 10 minutes. Allow cooling for a few minutes. Using an immersion blender, blitz the soup until smooth. Serve

33) BELL PEPPER AND MUSHROOM SOUP

Preparation Time: 45 minutes

Servings: 6

Ingredients:

- 3 tbsp olive oil
- 1 onion, chopped
- 1 large carrot, chopped
- 1 lb mixed bell peppers, chopped
- 1 cup cremini mushrooms, quartered
- 1 cup white mushrooms, quartered
- 6 cups vegetable broth
- ¼ cup chopped fresh parsley
- 1 tsp minced fresh thyme
- Salt and black pepper to taste

Directions:

- Heat the oil in a pot over medium heat. Place onion, carrot, and celery and cook for 5 minutes. Add in bell peppers and broth and stir. Bring to a boil, lower the heat, and simmer for 20 minutes. Adjust the seasoning with salt and black pepper. Serve in soup bowls topped with parsley and thyme

34) PUMPKIN CAYENNE SOUP

Preparation Time: 55 minutes

Servings: 6

Ingredients:

- 1 (2-pound) pumpkin, sliced
- 3 tbsp olive oil
- 1 tsp salt
- 2 red bell peppers
- 1 onion, halved
- 1 head garlic
- 6 cups water
- Zest and juice of 1 lime
- ¼ tsp cayenne pepper
- ½ tsp ground coriander
- ½ tsp ground cumin
- Toasted pumpkin seeds

Directions:

- Preheat oven to 350 F.
- Brush the pumpkin slices with oil and sprinkle with salt. Arrange the slices skin-side-down and on a greased baking dish and bake for 20 minutes. Brush the onion with oil. Cut the top of the garlic head and brush with oil.
- When the pumpkin is ready, add in bell peppers, onion, and garlic, and bake for another 10 minutes. Allow cooling.
- Take out the flesh from the pumpkin skin and transfer to a food processor. Cut the pepper roughly, peel and cut the onion, and remove the cloves from the garlic head. Transfer to the food processor and pour in the water, lime zest, and lime juice.
- Blend the soup until smooth. If it's very thick, add a bit of water to reach your desired consistency. Sprinkle with salt, cayenne, coriander, and cumin. Serve

35) ZUCCHINI CREAM SOUP WITH WALNUTS

Preparation Time: 45 minutes

Servings: 4

Ingredients:

- 3 zucchinis, chopped
- 2 tsp olive oil
- Sea salt and black pepper to taste
- 1 onion, diced
- 4 cups vegetable stock
- 3 tsp ground sage
- 3 tbsp nutritional yeast
- 1 cup non-dairy milk
- ¼ cup toasted walnuts

Directions:

- Heat the oil in a skillet and place zucchini, onion, salt, and pepper; cook for 5 minutes. Pour in vegetable stock and bring to a boil. Lower the heat and simmer for 15 minutes. Stir in sage, nutritional yeast, and milk. Purée the soup with a blender until smooth. Serve garnished with toasted walnuts and pepper

36) RAMEN SOUP

Preparation Time: 25 minutes

Servings: 4

Ingredients:

- 7 oz Japanese buckwheat noodles
- 4 tbsp sesame paste
- 1 cup canned pinto beans, drained
- 2 tbsp fresh cilantro, chopped
- 2 scallions, thinly sliced

Directions:

- In boiling salted water, add in the noodles and cook for 5 minutes over low heat. Remove a cup of the noodle water to a bowl and add in the sesame paste; stir until it has dissolved. Pour the sesame mix in the pot with the noodles, add in pinto beans, and stir until everything is hot. Serve topped with cilantro and scallions in individual bowls

37) BLACK-EYED PEA SOUP

Preparation Time: 45 minutes

Servings: 6

Ingredients:

- 2 carrots, chopped
- 1 onion, chopped
- 2 cups canned dried black-eyed peas
- 1 tbsp soy sauce
- 3 tsp dried thyme
- 1 tsp onion powder
- ½ tsp garlic powder
- Salt and black pepper to taste
- ¼ cup chopped pitted black olives

Directions:

- Place carrots, onion, black-eyed peas, 3 cups water, soy sauce, thyme, onion powder, garlic powder, and pepper in a pot. Bring to a boil, then reduce the heat to low. Cook for 20 minutes. Allow cooling for a few minutes. Transfer to a food processor and blend until smooth. Stir in black olives. Serve

The Plant-Based for Athlete

Vegetables and Side Dishes

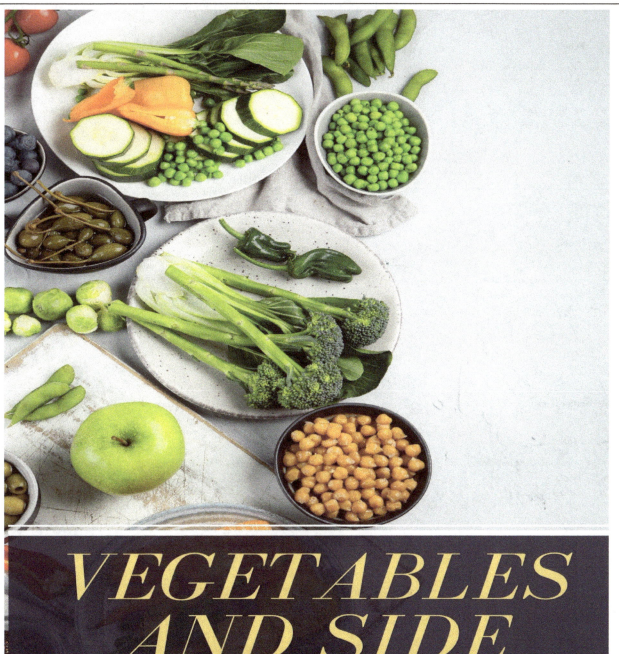

VEGETABLES AND SIDE DISHES

38) ROASTED KOHLRABI

Preparation Time: 30 minutes

Servings: 4

Ingredients:

- 1 pound kohlrabi bulbs, peeled and sliced
- 4 tbsp olive oil
- 1/2 tsp mustard seeds
- 1 tsp celery seeds
- 1 tsp dried marjoram
- 1 tsp granulated garlic, minced
- Sea salt and ground black pepper, to taste
- 2 tbsp nutritional yeast

Directions:

- Start by preheating your oven to 450 degrees F.
- Toss the kohlrabi with the olive oil and spices until well coated. Arrange the kohlrabi in a single layer on a parchment-lined roasting pan.
- Bake the kohlrabi in the preheated oven for about 15 minutes; stir them and continue to cook an additional 15 minutes.
- Sprinkle nutritional yeast over the warm kohlrabi and serve immediately. Enjoy

39) CAULIFLOWER WITH TAHINI SAUCE

Preparation Time: 10 minutes

Servings: 4

Ingredients:

- 1 cup water
- 2 pounds cauliflower florets
- Sea salt and ground black pepper, to taste
- 3 tbsp soy sauce
- 5 tbsp tahini
- 2 cloves garlic, minced
- 2 tbsp lemon juice

Directions:

- In a large saucepan, bring the water to a boil; then, add in the cauliflower and cook for about 6 minutes or until fork-tender; drain, season with salt and pepper and reserve.
- In a mixing bowl, thoroughly combine the soy sauce, tahini, garlic and lemon juice. Spoon the sauce over the cauliflower florets and serve.
- Enjoy

40) HERB CAULIFLOWER MASH

Preparation Time: 25 minutes

Servings: 4

Ingredients:

- 1 ½ pounds cauliflower florets
- 4 tbsp vegan butter
- 4 cloves garlic, sliced
- Sea salt and ground black pepper, to taste
- 1/4 cup plain oat milk, unsweetened
- 2 tbsp fresh parsley, roughly chopped

Directions:

- Steam the cauliflower florets for about 20 minutes; set it aside to cool.
- In a saucepan, melt the vegan butter over a moderately high heat; now, sauté the garlic for about 1 minute or until aromatic.
- Add the cauliflower florets to your food processor followed by the sautéed garlic, salt, black pepper and oat milk. Puree until everything is well incorporated.
- Garnish with fresh parsley leaves and serve hot. Enjoy

41) GARLIC AND HERB MUSHROOM SKILLET

Preparation Time: 10 minutes

Servings: 4

Ingredients:

- 4 tbsp vegan butter
- 1 ½ pounds oyster mushrooms halved
- 3 cloves garlic, minced
- 1 tsp dried oregano
- 1 tsp dried rosemary
- 1 tsp dried parsley flakes
- 1 tsp dried marjoram
- 1/2 cup dry white wine
- Kosher salt and ground black pepper, to taste

Directions:

- In a sauté pan, heat the olive oil over a moderately high heat.
- Now, sauté the mushrooms for 3 minutes or until they release the liquid. Add in the garlic and continue to cook for 30 seconds more or until aromatic.
- Stir in the spices and continue sautéing an additional 6 minutes, until your mushrooms are lightly browned.
- Enjoy

42) PAN-FRIED ASPARAGUS

Preparation Time: 10 minutes

Servings: 4

Ingredients:

- 4 tbsp vegan butter
- 1 ½ pounds asparagus spears, trimmed
- 1/2 tsp cumin seeds, ground
- 1/4 tsp bay leaf, ground
- Sea salt and ground black pepper, to taste
- 1 tsp fresh lime juice

Directions:

- Melt the vegan butter in a saucepan over medium-high heat.
- Sauté the asparagus for about 3 to 4 minutes, stirring periodically to promote even cooking.
- Add in the cumin seeds, bay leaf, salt and black pepper and continue to cook the asparagus for 2 minutes more until crisp-tender.
- Drizzle lime juice over the asparagus and serve warm. Enjoy

43) GINGERY CARROT MASH

Preparation Time: 25 minutes

Servings: 4

Ingredients:

- 2 pounds carrots, cut into rounds
- 2 tbsp olive oil
- 1 tsp ground cumin
- Salt ground black pepper, to taste
- 1/2 tsp cayenne pepper
- 1/2 tsp ginger, peeled and minced
- 1/2 cup whole milk

Directions:

- Begin by preheating your oven to 400 degrees F.
- Toss the carrots with the olive oil, cumin, salt, black pepper and cayenne pepper. Arrange them in a single layer on a parchment-lined roasting sheet.
- Roast the carrots in the preheated oven for about 20 minutes, until crisp-tender.
- Add the roasted carrots, ginger and milk to your food processor; puree the ingredients until everything is well blended.
- Enjoy

44) MEDITERRANEAN-STYLE ROASTED ARTICHOKES

Preparation Time: 50 minutes

Servings: 4

Ingredients:

- 4 artichokes, trimmed, tough outer leaves and chokes removed, halved
- 2 lemons, freshly squeezed
- 4 tbsp extra-virgin olive oil
- 4 cloves garlic, chopped
- 1 tsp fresh rosemary
- 1 tsp fresh basil
- 1 tsp fresh parsley
- 1 tsp fresh oregano
- Flaky sea salt and ground black pepper, to taste
- 1 tsp red pepper flakes
- 1 tsp paprika

Directions:

- Start by preheating your oven to 395 degrees F. Rub the lemon juice all over the entire surface of your artichokes.
- In a small mixing bowl, thoroughly combine the garlic with herbs and spices
- Place the artichoke halves in a parchment-lined baking dish, cut-side-up. Brush the artichokes evenly with the olive oil. Fill the cavities with the garlic/herb mixture.
- Bake for about 20 minutes. Now, cover them with aluminum foil and bake for a further 30 minutes. Serve warm and enjoy

45) THAI-STYLE BRAISED KALE

Preparation Time: 10 minutes

Servings: 4

Ingredients:

- 1 cup water
- 1 ½ pounds kale, tough stems and ribs removed, torn into pieces
- 2 tbsp sesame oil
- 1 tsp fresh garlic, pressed
- 1 tsp ginger, peeled and minced
- 1 Thai chili, chopped
- 1/2 tsp turmeric powder
- 1/2 cup coconut milk
- Kosher salt and ground black pepper, to taste

Directions:

- In a large saucepan, bring the water to a rapid boil. Add in the kale and let it cook until bright, about 3 minutes. Drain, rinse and squeeze dry.
- Wipe the saucepan with paper towels and preheat the sesame oil over a moderate heat. Once hot, cook the garlic, ginger and chili for approximately 1 minute or so, until fragrant.
- Add in the kale and turmeric powder and continue to cook for a further 1 minute or until heated through.
- Gradually pour in the coconut milk, salt and black pepper; continue to simmer until the liquid has thickened. Taste, adjust the seasonings and serve hot. Enjoy

46) SILKY KOHLRABI PUREE

Preparation Time: 30 minutes

Servings: 4

Ingredients:

- 1 ½ pounds kohlrabi, peeled and cut into pieces
- 4 tbsp vegan butter
- Sea salt and freshly ground black pepper, to taste
- 1/2 tsp cumin seeds
- 1/2 tsp coriander seeds
- 1/2 cup soy milk
- 1 tsp fresh dill
- 1 tsp fresh parsley

Directions:

- Cook the kohlrabi in boiling salted water until soft, about 30 minutes; drain.
- Puree the kohlrabi with the vegan butter, salt, black pepper, cumin seeds and coriander seeds.
- Puree the ingredients with an immersion blender, gradually adding the milk. Top with fresh dill and parsley. Enjoy

47) CREAMY SAUTÉED SPINACH

Preparation Time: 15 minutes

Servings: 4

Ingredients:

- 2 tbsp vegan butter
- 1 onion, chopped
- 1 tsp garlic, minced
- 1 ½ cups vegetable broth
- 2 pounds spinach, torn into pieces
- Sea salt and ground black pepper, to taste
- 1/4 tsp dried dill
- 1/4 tsp mustard seeds
- 1/2 tsp celery seeds
- 1 tsp cayenne pepper
- 1/2 cup oat milk

Directions:

- In a saucepan, melt the vegan butter over medium-high heat.
- Then, sauté the onion for about 3 minutes or until tender and translucent. Then, sauté the garlic for about 1 minute until aromatic.
- Add in the broth and spinach and bring to a boil.
- Turn the heat to a simmer. Add in the spices and continue to cook for 5 minutes longer.
- Add in the milk and continue to cook for 5 minutes more. Enjoy

48) ROASTED CARROTS WITH HERBS

Preparation Time: 25 minute

Servings: 4

Ingredients:

- 2 pounds carrots, trimmed and halved lengthwise
- 4 tbsp olive oil
- 1 tsp granulated garlic
- 1 tsp paprika
- Sea salt and freshly ground black pepper
- 2 tbsp fresh cilantro, chopped
- 2 tbsp fresh parsley, chopped
- 2 tbsp fresh chives, chopped

Directions:

- Start by preheating your oven to 400 degrees F.
- Toss the carrots with the olive oil, granulated garlic, paprika, salt and black pepper. Arrange them in a single layer on a parchment-lined roasting sheet.
- Roast the carrots in the preheated oven for about 20 minutes, until fork-tender.
- Toss the carrots with the fresh herbs and serve immediately. Enjoy

49) BRAISED GREEN BEANS

Preparation Time: 15 minutes

Servings: 4

Ingredients:

- 4 tbsp olive oil
- 1 carrot, cut into matchsticks
- 1 ½ pounds green beans, trimmed
- 4 garlic cloves, peeled
- 1 bay laurel
- 1 ½ cups vegetable broth
- Sea salt and ground black pepper, to taste
- 1 lemon, cut into wedges

Directions:

- Heat the olive oil in a saucepan over medium flame. Once hot, fry the carrots and green beans for about 5 minutes, stirring periodically to promote even cooking.
- Add in the garlic and bay laurel and continue sautéing an additional 1 minute or until fragrant.
- Add in the broth, salt and black pepper and continue to simmer, covered, for about 9 minutes or until the green beans are tender.
- Taste, adjust the seasonings and serve with lemon wedges. Enjoy

Lunch

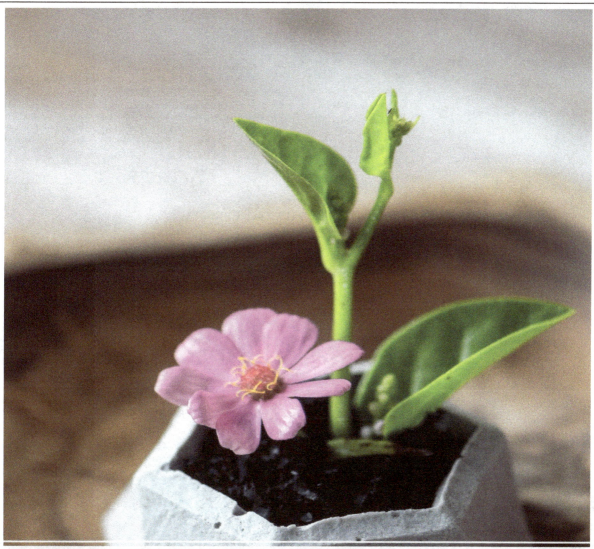

LUNCH

50) JALAPEÑO QUINOA BOWL WITH LIMA BEANS

Preparation Time: 30 minutes

Servings: 4

Ingredients:

- 1 tbsp olive oil
- 1 lb extra firm tofu, cubed
- Salt and black pepper to taste
- 1 medium yellow onion, finely diced
- ½ cup cauliflower florets
- 1 jalapeño pepper, minced
- 2 garlic cloves, minced
- 1 tbsp red chili powder
- 1 tsp cumin powder
- 1 (8 oz) can sweet corn kernels
- 1 (8 oz) can lima beans, rinsed
- 1 cup quick-cooking quinoa
- 1 (14 oz) can diced tomatoes
- 2 ½ cups vegetable broth
- 1 cup grated plant-based cheddar
- 2 tbsp chopped fresh cilantro
- 2 limes, cut into wedges
- 1 avocado, pitted, sliced, and peeled

Directions:

- Heat olive oil in a pot and cook the tofu until golden brown, 5 minutes. Season with salt, pepper, and mix in onion, cauliflower, and jalapeño pepper. Cook until the vegetables soften, 3 minutes.
- Stir in garlic, chili powder, and cumin powder; cook for 1 minute. Mix in sweet corn kernels, lima beans, quinoa, tomatoes, and vegetable broth. Simmer until the quinoa absorbs all the liquid, 10 minutes. Fluff quinoa. Top with the plant-based cheddar cheese, cilantro, lime wedges, and avocado. Serve

51) AVOCADO COCONUT PIE

Preparation Time: 80 minutes

Servings: 4

Ingredients:

- Piecrust:
- 1 tbsp flax seed powder + 3 tbsp water
- 1 cup coconut flour
- 4 tbsp chia seeds
- 1 tbsp psyllium husk powder
- 1 tsp baking soda
- 1 pinch salt
- 3 tbsp coconut oil
- 4 tbsp water
- Filling:
- 2 ripe avocados, chopped
- 1 cup tofu mayonnaise
- 3 tbsp flax seed powder + 9 tbsp water
- 2 tbsp fresh parsley, chopped
- 1 jalapeno, finely chopped
- ½ tsp onion powder
- ¼ tsp salt
- ½ cup cream cheese
- 1 ¼ cups grated plant-based Parmesan

Directions:

- In 2 separate bowls, mix the different portions of flax seed powder with the respective quantity of water. Allow absorbing for 5 minutes.
- Preheat oven to 350 F. In a food processor, add the piecrust ingredients and the smaller portion of the vegan "flax egg." Blend until the resulting dough forms into a ball. Line a springform pan with parchment paper and spread the dough in the pan. Bake for 10-15 minutes.
- Put the avocado in a bowl and add the tofu mayonnaise, remaining vegan "flax egg," parsley, jalapeno, onion powder, salt, cream cheese, and plant-based Parmesan. Combine well. Remove the piecrust when ready and fill with the creamy mixture. Bake for 35 minutes. Cool before slicing and serving

52) GREEN AVOCADO CARBONARA

Preparation Time: 30 minutes

Servings: 4

Ingredients:

- 8 tbsp flax seed powder
- 1 ½ cups cashew cream cheese
- 5 ½ tbsp psyllium husk powder
- 1 avocado, chopped
- 1 ¾ cups coconut cream
- Juice of ½ lemon
- 1 tsp onion powder
- ½ tsp garlic powder
- ¼ cup olive oil
- Salt and black pepper to taste
- ½ cup grated plant-based Parmesan
- 4 tbsp toasted pecans

Directions:

- Preheat oven to 300 F.
- In a medium bowl, mix the flax seed powder with 1 ½ cups water and allow sitting to thicken for 5 minutes. Add the cashew cream cheese, salt, and psyllium husk powder. Whisk until smooth batter forms. Line a baking sheet with parchment paper, pour in the batter, and cover with another parchment paper. Use a rolling pin to flatten the dough into the sheet. Bake for 10-12 minutes. Remove, take off the parchment papers and use a sharp knife to slice the pasta into thin strips lengthwise. Cut each piece into halves, pour into a bowl, and set aside.
- In a blender, combine avocado, coconut cream, lemon juice, onion powder, and garlic powder; puree until smooth. Pour the olive oil over the pasta and stir to coat properly. Pour the avocado sauce on top and mix. Season with salt and black pepper. Divide the pasta into serving plates, garnish with Parmesan cheese and pecans, and serve immediately

53) MUSHROOM AND GREEN BEAN BIRYANI

Preparation Time: 50 minutes

Servings: 4

Ingredients:

- 1 cup brown rice
- 3 tbsp plant butter
- 3 medium white onions, chopped
- 6 garlic cloves, minced
- 1 tsp ginger puree
- 1 tbsp turmeric powder + for dusting
- ¼ tsp cinnamon powder
- 2 tsp garam masala
- ½ tsp cardamom powder
- ½ tsp cayenne powder
- ½ tsp cumin powder
- 1 tsp smoked paprika
- 3 large tomatoes, diced
- 2 green chilies, minced
- 1 tbsp tomato puree
- 1 cup chopped cremini mushrooms
- 1 cup chopped mustard greens
- 1 cup plant-based yogurt

Directions:

- Melt the butter in a large pot and sauté the onions until softened, 3 minutes. Mix in the garlic, ginger, turmeric, cardamom powder, garam masala, cardamom powder, cayenne pepper, cumin powder, paprika, and salt. Stir-fry for 1-2 minutes.
- Stir in the tomatoes, green chili, tomato puree, and mushrooms. Once boiling, mix in the rice and cover with water. Cover the pot and cook over medium heat until the liquid absorbs and the rice is tender, 15-20 minutes. Open the lid and fluff in the mustard greens and half of the parsley. Dish the food, top with the coconut yogurt, garnish with the remaining parsley, and serve warm

54) MUSHROOM LETTUCE WRAPS

Preparation Time: 25 minutes

Servings: 4

Ingredients:

- 2 tbsp plant butter
- 4 oz baby Bella mushrooms, sliced
- 1 ½ lb tofu, crumbled
- 1 iceberg lettuce, leaves extracted
- 1 cup grated plant-based cheddar
- 1 large tomato, sliced

Directions:

- Melt the plant butter in a skillet, add in mushrooms and sauté until browned and tender, about 6 minutes. Transfer to a plate. Add the tofu to the skillet and cook until brown, about 10 minutes. Spoon the tofu and mushrooms into the lettuce leaves, sprinkle with the plant-based cheddar cheese, and share the tomato slices on top. Serve the burger immediately

55) CLASSIC GARLICKY RICE

Preparation Time: 20 minutes

Servings: 4

Ingredients:

- 4 tbsp olive oil
- 4 cloves garlic, chopped
- 1 ½ cups white rice
- 2 ½ cups vegetable broth

Directions:

- In a saucepan, heat the olive oil over a moderately high flame. Add in the garlic and sauté for about 1 minute or until aromatic.
- Add in the rice and broth. Bring to a boil; immediately turn the heat to a gentle simmer.
- Cook for about 15 minutes or until all the liquid has absorbed. Fluff the rice with a fork, season with salt and pepper and serve hot

56) BROWN RICE WITH VEGETABLES AND TOFU

Preparation Time: 45 minutes

Servings: 4

Ingredients:

- 4 tsp sesame seeds
- 2 spring garlic stalks, minced
- 1 cup spring onions, chopped
- 1 carrot, trimmed and sliced
- 1 celery rib, sliced
- 1/4 cup dry white wine
- 10 ounces tofu, cubed
- 1 ½ cups long-grain brown rice, rinsed thoroughly
- 2 tbsp soy sauce
- 2 tbsp tahini
- 1 tbsp lemon juice

Directions:

- In a wok or large saucepan, heat 2 tsp of the sesame oil over medium-high heat. Now, cook the garlic, onion, carrot and celery for about 3 minutes, stirring periodically to ensure even cooking.
- Add the wine to deglaze the pan and push the vegetables to one side of the wok. Add in the remaining sesame oil and fry the tofu for 8 minutes, stirring occasionally.
- Bring 2 ½ cups of water to a boil over medium-high heat. Bring to a simmer and cook the rice for about 30 minutes or until it is tender; fluff the rice and stir it with the soy sauce and tahini.
- Stir the vegetables and tofu into the hot rice; add a few drizzles of the fresh lemon juice and serve warm. Enjoy

57) AMARANTH PORRIDGE

Preparation Time: 35 minutes

Servings: 4

Ingredients:

- 3 cups water
- 1 cup amaranth
- 1/2 cup coconut milk
- 4 tbsp agave syrup
- A pinch of kosher salt
- A pinch of grated nutmeg

Directions:

- Bring the water to a boil over medium-high heat; add in the amaranth and turn the heat to a simmer.
- Let it cook for about 30 minutes, stirring periodically to prevent the amaranth from sticking to the bottom of the pan.
- Stir in the remaining ingredients and continue to cook for 1 to 2 minutes more until cooked through. Enjoy

58) MUM'S AROMATIC RICE

Preparation Time: 20 minutes

Servings: 4

Ingredients:

- 3 tbsp olive oil
- 1 tsp garlic, minced
- 1 tsp dried oregano
- 1 tsp dried rosemary
- 1 bay leaf
- 1 ½ cups white rice
- 2 ½ cups vegetable broth
- Sea salt and cayenne pepper, to taste

Directions:

- In a saucepan, heat the olive oil over a moderately high flame. Add in the garlic, oregano, rosemary and bay leaf; sauté for about 1 minute or until aromatic.
- Add in the rice and broth. Bring to a boil; immediately turn the heat to a gentle simmer.
- Cook for about 15 minutes or until all the liquid has absorbed. Fluff the rice with a fork, season with salt and pepper and serve immediately.
- Enjoy

59) EVERYDAY SAVORY GRITS

Preparation Time: 35 minutes

Servings: 4

Ingredients:

- 2 tbsp vegan butter
- 1 sweet onion, chopped
- 1 tsp garlic, minced
- 4 cups water
- 1 cup stone-ground grits
- Sea salt and cayenne pepper, to taste

Directions:

- In a saucepan, melt the vegan butter over medium-high heat. Once hot, cook the onion for about 3 minutes or until tender.
- Add in the garlic and continue to sauté for 30 seconds more or until aromatic; reserve.
- Bring the water to a boil over a moderately high heat. Stir in the grits, salt and pepper. Turn the heat to a simmer, cover and continue to cook, for about 30 minutes or until cooked through.
- Stir in the sautéed mixture and serve warm. Enjoy

60) GREEK-STYLE BARLEY SALAD

Preparation Time: 35 minutes

Servings: 4

Ingredients:

- 1 cup pearl barley
- 2 ¾ cups vegetable broth
- 2 tbsp apple cider vinegar
- 4 tbsp extra-virgin olive oil
- 2 bell peppers, seeded and diced
- 1 shallot, chopped
- 2 ounces sun-dried tomatoes in oil, chopped
- 1/2 green olives, pitted and sliced
- 2 tbsp fresh cilantro, roughly chopped

Directions:

- Bring the barley and broth to a boil over medium-high heat; now, turn the heat to a simmer.
- Continue to simmer for about 30 minutes until all the liquid has absorbed; fluff with a fork.
- Toss the barley with the vinegar, olive oil, peppers, shallots, sun-dried tomatoes and olives; toss to combine well.
- Garnish with fresh cilantro and serve at room temperature or well-chilled. Enjoy

61) SWEET MAIZE MEAL PORRIDGE

Preparation Time: 15 minutes

Servings: 2

Ingredients:

- 2 cups water
- 1/2 cup maize meal
- 1/4 tsp ground allspice
- 1/4 tsp salt
- 2 tbsp brown sugar
- 2 tbsp almond butter

Directions:

- In a saucepan, bring the water to a boil; then, gradually add in the maize meal and turn the heat to a simmer.
- Add in the ground allspice and salt. Let it cook for 10 minutes.
- Add in the brown sugar and almond butter and gently stir to combine. Enjoy

62) FOCACCIA WITH MIXED MUSHROOMS

Preparation Time: 35 minutes

Servings: 4

Ingredients:

- 2 tbsp flax seed powder
- ½ cup tofu mayonnaise
- ¾ cup almond flour
- 1 tbsp psyllium husk powder
- 1 tsp baking powder
- 2 oz mixed mushrooms, sliced
- 1 tbsp plant-based basil pesto
- 2 tbsp olive oil
- Salt and black pepper to taste
- ½ cup coconut cream
- ¾ cup grated plant-based Parmesan

Directions:

- Preheat oven to 350 F.
- Combine flax seed powder with 6 tbsp water and allow sitting to thicken for 5 minutes. Whisk in tofu mayonnaise, almond flour, psyllium husk powder, baking powder, and salt. Allow sitting for 5 minutes. Pour the batter into a baking sheet and spread out with a spatula. Bake for 10 minutes.
- In a bowl, mix mushrooms with pesto, olive oil, salt, and black pepper. Remove the crust from the oven and spread the coconut cream on top. Add the mushroom mixture and plant-based Parmesan cheese. Bake the pizza further until the cheese has melted, 5-10 minutes. Slice and serve with salad

63) SEITAN CAKES WITH BROCCOLI MASH

Preparation Time: 30 minutes

Servings: 4

Ingredients:

- 1 tbsp flax seed powder
- 1 ½ lb crumbled seitan
- ½ white onion
- 2 oz olive oil
- 1 lb broccoli
- 5 oz cold plant butter
- 2 oz grated plant-based Parmesan
- 4 oz plant butter, room temperature
- 2 tbsp lemon juice

Directions:

- Preheat oven to 220 F. In a bowl, mix the flax seed powder with 3 tbsp water and allow sitting to thicken for 5 minutes. When the vegan "flax egg" is ready, add in crumbled seitan, white onion, salt, and pepper. Mix and mold out 6-8 cakes out of the mixture. Melt plant butter in a skillet and fry the patties on both sides until golden brown. Remove onto a wire rack to cool slightly.
- Pour salted water into a pot, bring to a boil, and add in broccoli. Cook until the broccoli is tender but not too soft. Drain and transfer to a bowl. Add in cold plant butter, plant-based Parmesan, salt, and pepper. Puree the ingredients until smooth and creamy. Set aside. Mix the soft plant butter with lemon juice, salt, and pepper in a bowl. Serve the seitan cakes with the broccoli mash and lemon butter

64) SPICY CHEESE WITH TOFU BALLS

Preparation Time: 40 minutes

Servings: 4

Ingredients:

- 1/3 cup tofu mayonnaise
- ¼ cup pickled jalapenos
- 1 tsp paprika powder
- 1 tbsp mustard powder
- 1 pinch cayenne pepper
- 4 oz grated plant-based cheddar
- 1 tbsp flax seed powder
- 2 ½ cup crumbled tofu
- 2 tbsp plant butter

Directions:

- In a bowl, mix tofu mayonnaise, jalapeños, paprika, mustard powder, cayenne powder, and plant-based cheddar cheese; set aside. In another bowl, combine flax seed powder with 3 tbsp water and allow absorbing for 5 minutes. Add the vegan "flax egg" to the cheese mixture, crumbled tofu, salt, and pepper and combine well. Form meatballs out of the mix. Melt plant butter in a skillet and fry the tofu balls until browned. Serve the tofu balls with roasted cauliflower mash

65) QUINOA ANDVEGGIE BURGERS

Preparation Time: 35 minutes

Servings: 4

Ingredients:

- 1 cup quick-cooking quinoa
- 1 tbsp olive oil
- 1 shallot, chopped
- 2 tbsp chopped fresh celery
- 1 garlic clove, minced
- 1 (15 oz) can pinto beans, drained
- 2 tbsp whole-wheat flour
- ¼ cup chopped fresh basil
- 2 tbsp pure maple syrup
- 4 whole-grain hamburger buns, split
- 4 small lettuce leaves for topping
- ½ cup tofu mayonnaise for topping

Directions:

- Cook the quinoa with 2 cups of water in a medium pot until the liquid absorbs, 10 to 15 minutes. Heat the olive oil in a medium skillet over medium heat and sauté the shallot, celery, and garlic until softened and fragrant, 3 minutes.
- Transfer the quinoa and shallot mixture to a medium bowl and add the pinto beans, flour, basil, maple syrup, salt, and black pepper. Mash and mold 4 patties out of the mixture and set aside.
- Heat a grill pan to medium heat and lightly grease with cooking spray. Cook the patties on both sides until light brown, compacted, and cooked through, 10 minutes. Place the patties between the burger buns and top with the lettuce and tofu mayonnaise. Serve

66) BAKED TOFU WITH ROASTED PEPPERS

Preparation Time: 20 minutes

Servings: 4

Ingredients:

- 3 oz cashew cream cheese
- ¾ cup tofu mayonnaise
- 2 oz cucumber, diced
- 1 large tomato, chopped
- 2 tsp dried parsley
- 4 medium orange bell peppers
- 2 ½ cups cubed tofu
- 1 tbsp melted plant butter
- 1 tsp dried basil

Directions:

- Preheat the oven's broiler to 450 F and line a baking sheet with parchment paper. In a salad bowl, combine cashew cream cheese, tofu mayonnaise, cucumber, tomato, salt, pepper, and parsley. Refrigerate.
- Arrange the bell peppers and tofu on the baking sheet, drizzle with melted plant butter, and season with basil, salt, and pepper. Bake for 10-15 minutes or until the peppers have charred lightly and the tofu browned. Remove from the oven and serve with the salad

67) ZOODLE BOLOGNESE

Preparation Time: 45 minutes

Servings: 4

Ingredients:

- 3 oz olive oil
- 1 white onion, chopped
- 1 garlic clove, minced
- 3 oz carrots, chopped
- 3 cups crumbled tofu
- 2 tbsp tomato paste
- 1 ½ cups crushed tomatoes
- Salt and black pepper to taste
- 1 tbsp dried basil
- 1 tbsp vegan Worcestershire sauce
- 2 lb zucchini, spiralized
- 2 tbsp plant butter

Directions:

- Pour olive oil into a saucepan and heat over medium heat. Add in onion, garlic, and carrots and sauté for 3 minutes or until the onions are soft and the carrots caramelized. Pour in tofu, tomato paste, tomatoes, salt, pepper, basil, and Worcestershire sauce. Stir and cook for 15 minutes. Mix in some water if the mixture is too thick and simmer further for 20 minutes. Melt plant butter in a skillet and toss in the zoodles quickly, about 1 minute. Season with salt and black pepper. Divide into serving plates and spoon the Bolognese on top. Serve immediately

68) ZUCCHINI BOATS WITH VEGAN CHEESE

Preparation Time: 40 minutes

Servings: 2

Ingredients:

- 1 medium-sized zucchini
- 4 tbsp plant butter
- 2 garlic cloves, minced
- 1 ½ oz baby kale
- Salt and black pepper to taste
- 2 tbsp unsweetened tomato sauce
- 1 cup grated plant-based mozzarella
- Olive oil for drizzling

Directions:

- Preheat oven to 375 F.
- Use a knife to slice the zucchini in halves and scoop out the pulp with a spoon into a plate. Keep the flesh. Grease a baking sheet with cooking spray and place the zucchini boats on top. Put the plant butter in a skillet and melt over medium heat.
- Sauté the garlic for 1 minute. Add in kale and zucchini pulp. Cook until the kale wilts; season with salt and black pepper. Spoon tomato sauce into the boats and spread to coat the bottom evenly. Then, spoon the kale mixture into the zucchinis and sprinkle with the plant-based mozzarella cheese. Bake for 20-25 minutes. Serve immediately

69) ROASTED BUTTERNUT SQUASH WITH CHIMICHURRI

Preparation Time: 15 minutes

Servings: 4

Ingredients:

- Zest and juice of 1 lemon
- ½ medium red bell pepper, chopped
- 1 jalapeno pepper, chopped
- 1 cup olive oil
- ½ cup chopped fresh parsley
- 2 garlic cloves, minced
- 1 lb butternut squash
- 1 tbsp plant butter, melted
- 3 tbsp toasted pine nuts

Directions:

- In a bowl, add the lemon zest and juice, red bell pepper, jalapeno, olive oil, parsley, garlic, salt, and black pepper. Use an immersion blender to grind the ingredients until your desired consistency is achieved; set aside the chimichurri.
- Slice the butternut squash into rounds and remove the seeds. Drizzle with the plant butter and season with salt and black pepper. Preheat a grill pan over medium heat and cook the squash for 2 minutes on each side or until browned. Remove the squash to serving plates, scatter the pine nuts on top, and serve with the chimichurri and red cabbage salad

70) BLACK BEAN BURGERS WITH BBQ SAUCE

Preparation Time: 20 minutes

Servings: 4

- Salt and black pepper to taste
- 4 whole-grain hamburger buns, split
- For topping:
- Red onion slices
- Tomato slices
- Fresh basil leaves
- Additional barbecue sauce

Directions:

- In a medium bowl, mash the black beans and mix in the flour, oats, basil, barbecue sauce, garlic salt, and black pepper until well combined. Mold 4 patties out of the mixture and set aside.
- Heat a grill pan to medium heat and lightly grease with cooking spray. Cook the bean patties on both sides until light brown and cooked through, 10 minutes. Place the patties between the burger buns and top with the onions, tomatoes, basil, and some barbecue sauce. Serve warm

71) CREAMY BRUSSELS SPROUTS BAKE

Preparation Time: 26 minutes

Servings: 4

- 1 ¼ cups coconut cream
- 10 oz grated plant-based mozzarella
- ¼ cup grated plant-based Parmesan
- Salt and black pepper to taste

Directions:

- Preheat oven to 400 F.
- Melt the plant butter in a large skillet over medium heat and fry the tempeh cubes until browned on both sides, about 6 minutes. Remove onto a plate and set aside. Pour the Brussels sprouts and garlic into the skillet and sauté until fragrant.
- Mix in coconut cream and simmer for 4 minutes. Add tempeh cubes and combine well. Pour the sauté into a baking dish, sprinkle with plant-based mozzarella cheese, and plant-based Parmesan cheese. Bake for 10 minutes or until golden brown on top. Serve with tomato salad

72) BAKED CHEESY SPAGHETTI SQUASH

Preparation Time: 40 minutes

Servings: 4

Ingredients:

- 2 lb spaghetti squash
- 1 tbsp coconut oil
- Salt and black pepper to taste
- 2 tbsp melted plant butter
- ½ tbsp garlic powder
- 1/5 tsp chili powder
- 1 cup coconut cream
- 2 oz cashew cream cheese
- 1 cup plant-based mozzarella
- 2 oz grated plant-based Parmesan
- 2 tbsp fresh cilantro, chopped
- Olive oil for drizzling

Directions:

- Preheat oven to 350 F.
- Cut the squash in halves lengthwise and spoon out the seeds and fiber. Place on a baking dish, brush with coconut oil, and season with salt and pepper. Bake for 30 minutes. Remove and use two forks to shred the flesh into strands.
- Empty the spaghetti strands into a bowl and mix with plant butter, garlic and chili powders, coconut cream, cream cheese, half of the plant-based mozzarella and plant-based Parmesan cheeses. Spoon the mixture into the squash cups and sprinkle with the remaining mozzarella cheese. Bake further for 5 minutes. Sprinkle with cilantro and drizzle with some oil. Serve

73) KALE AND MUSHROOM PIEROGIS

Preparation Time: 45 minutes

Servings: 4

Ingredients:

- Stuffing:
- 2 tbsp plant butter
- 2 garlic cloves, finely chopped
- 1 small red onion, finely chopped
- 3 oz baby Bella mushrooms, sliced
- 2 oz fresh kale
- ½ tsp salt
- ¼ tsp freshly ground black pepper
- ½ cup dairy-free cream cheese
- 2 oz plant-based Parmesan, grated
- Pierogi:
- 1 tbsp flax seed powder
- ½ cup almond flour
- 4 tbsp coconut flour
- ½ tsp salt
- 1 tsp baking powder
- 1 ½ cups grated plant-based Parmesan
- 5 tbsp plant butter
- Olive oil for brushing

Directions:

- Put the plant butter in a skillet and melt over medium heat, then add and sauté the garlic, red onion, mushrooms, and kale until the mushrooms brown. Season the mixture with salt and black pepper and reduce the heat to low. Stir in the cream cheese and plant-based Parmesan cheese and simmer for 1 minute. Turn the heat off and set the filling aside to cool.
- Make the pierogis: In a small bowl, mix the flax seed powder with 3 tbsp water and allow sitting for 5 minutes. In a bowl, combine almond flour, coconut flour, salt, and baking powder. Put a small pan over low heat, add, and melt the plant-based Parmesan cheese and plant butter while stirring continuously until smooth batter forms. Turn the heat off.
- Pour the vegan "flax egg" into the cream mixture, continue stirring while adding the flour mixture until a firm dough forms. Mold the dough into four balls, place on a chopping board, and use a rolling pin to flatten each into ½ inch thin round pieces. Spread a generous amount of stuffing on one-half of each dough, then fold over the filling, and seal the dough with your fingers. Brush with olive oil, place on a baking sheet, and bake for 20 minutes at 380 F. Serve with salad

74) VEGAN MUSHROOM PIZZA

Preparation Time: 35 minutes

Servings: 4

Ingredients:

- 2 tsp plant butter
- 1 cup chopped button mushrooms
- ½ cup sliced mixed bell peppers
- Salt and black pepper to taste
- 1 pizza crust
- 1 cup tomato sauce
- 1 cup plant-based Parmesan cheese
- 5-6 basil leaves

Directions:

- Melt plant butter in a skillet and sauté mushrooms and bell peppers for 10 minutes until softened. Season with salt and black pepper. Put the pizza crust on a pizza pan, spread the tomato sauce all over, and scatter vegetables evenly on top. Sprinkle with plant-based Parmesan cheese. Bake for 20 minutes until the cheese has melted. Garnish with basil and serve

Dinner

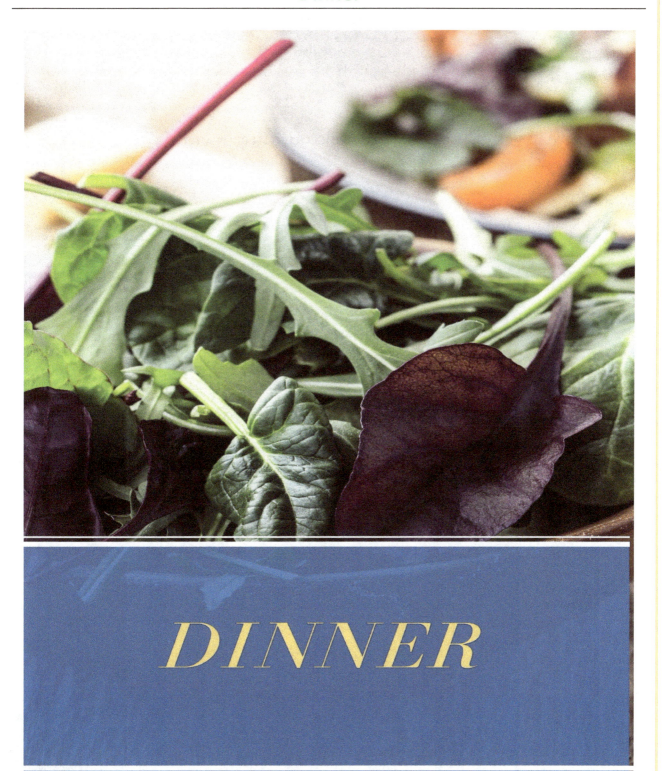

DINNER

75) PARSLEY CARROTS AND PARSNIPS

Preparation Time: 25 minutes

Servings: 4

Ingredients:

- 2 tbsp plant butter
- ½ lb carrots, cut lengthways
- ½ lb parsnips, cut lengthways
- Salt and black pepper to taste
- ½ cup Port wine
- ¼ cup chopped fresh parsley

Directions:

- Melt the butter in a skillet over medium heat. Place in carrots and parsnips and cook for 5 minutes, stirring occasionally. Sprinkle with salt and pepper. Pour in Port wine and ¼ cup water. Lower the heat and simmer for 15 minutes. Uncover and increase the heat. Cook until a syrupy sauce forms. Remove to a bowl and serve garnished with parsley

76) SESAME ROASTED BROCCOLI WITH BROWN RICE

Preparation Time: 30 minutes

Servings: 4

Ingredients:

- 1 head broccoli, cut into florets
- 2 tbsp olive oil
- ¾ cup pure date sugar
- ⅔ cup water
- ⅓ cup apple cider vinegar
- 1 tbsp ketchup
- ¼ cup soy sauce
- 2 tbsp corn-starch
- 4 cups cooked brown rice
- 2 scallions, chopped
- Sesame seeds

Directions:

- Preheat oven to 420 F. Line with parchment paper a baking sheet. Coat the broccoli with oil in a bowl. Spread on the baking sheet and roast for 20 minutes, turning once.
- Add the sugar, water, vinegar, and ketchup to a skillet and bring to a boil. Lower the heat and simmer for 5 minutes. In a bowl, whisk the soy sauce with corn-starch and pour it into the skillet. Stir for 2-4 minutes. Once the broccoli is ready, transfer into the skillet and toss to combine. Share the rice into 4 bowls and top with the broccoli. Serve garnished with scallions and sesame seeds

77) MATCHA-INFUSED TOFU RICE

Servings: 4

- 2 cups snow peas, cut diagonally
- 1 tbsp fresh lemon juice
- 1 tsp grated lemon zest
- Salt and black pepper to taste

Directions:

- Boil 3 cups water in a pot. Place in the tea bags and turn the heat off. Let sit for 7 minutes. Discard the bags. Wash the rice and put it into the tea. Cook for 20 minutes over medium heat. Drain and set aside.
- Heat the oil in a skillet over medium heat. Fry the tofu for 5 minutes until golden. Stir in green onions and snow peas and cook for another 3 minutes. Mix in lemon juice and lemon zest. Place the rice in a serving bowl and mix in the tofu mixture. Adjust the seasoning with salt and pepper. Serve right away

78) CHINESE FRIED RICE

Servings: 4

- 3 green onions, minced
- 3 ½ cups cooked brown rice
- 1 cup frozen peas, thawed
- 3 tbsp soy sauce
- 2 tsp dry white wine
- 1 tbsp toasted sesame oil

Directions:

- Heat the oil in a skillet over medium heat. Place in onion, carrot, and broccoli, sauté for 5 minutes until tender. Add in garlic, ginger, and green onions and sauté for another 3 minutes. Stir in rice, peas, soy sauce, and white wine and cook for 5 minutes. Add in sesame oil, toss to combine. Serve right away

79) PEPPERED PINTO BEANS

Preparation Time: 30 minutes

Servings: 6

Ingredients:
- 1 serrano pepper, cut into strips
- 1 red bell pepper, cut into strips
- 1 green bell pepper, cut into strips
- 1 onion, chopped
- 2 carrots, chopped
- 2 garlic cloves, minced
- 3 (15-oz) cans pinto beans
- 18-ounce bottle barbecue sauce
- ½ tsp chipotle powder

Directions:
- In a blender, place the serrano and bell peppers, onion, carrot, and garlic. Pulse until well mixed.
- Place the mixture in a pot with the beans, BBQ sauce, and chipotle powder. Cook for 15 minutes. Season with salt and pepper. Serve warm

80) BLACK-EYED PEAS WITH SUN-DRIED TOMATOES

Preparation Time: 35 minutes

Servings: 4

Ingredients:
- 1 cup black-eyed peas, soaked overnight
- ¼ cup sun-dried tomatoes, chopped
- 2 tbsp olive oil
- 2 tsp ground chipotle pepper
- 1 ½ tsp ground cumin
- 1 ½ tsp onion powder
- 1 tsp dried oregano
- ¾ tsp garlic powder
- ½ tsp smoked paprika

Directions:
- Place the black-eyed peas in a pot and add 2 cups of water, olive oil, chipotle pepper, cumin, onion powder, oregano, garlic powder, salt, and paprika. Cook for 20 minutes over medium heat. Mix in sun-dried tomatoes, let sit for a few minutes and serve

81) VEGETARIAN QUINOA CURRY

Preparation Time: 35 minutes

Servings: 4

Ingredients:
- 4 tsp olive oil
- 1 onion, chopped
- 2 tbsp curry powder
- 1 ½ cups quinoa
- 1 cup canned diced tomatoes
- 4 cups chopped spinach
- ½ cup non-dairy milk
- 2 tbsp soy sauce
- Salt to taste

Directions:
- Heat the oil in a pot over medium heat. Sauté the onion and ginger for 3 minutes until tender. Pour in curry powder, quinoa, and 3 cups of water. Bring to a boil, then lower the heat and simmer for 15-20 minutes. Mix in tomatoes, spinach, milk, soy sauce, and salt. Simmer for an additional 3 minutes

82) ALFREDO RICE WITH GREEN BEANS

Preparation Time: 25 minutes

Servings: 3

Ingredients:
- 1 cup Alfredo arugula vegan pesto
- 1 cup frozen green beans, thawed
- 2 cups brown rice

Directions:
- Cook the rice in salted water in a pot over medium heat for 20 minutes. Drain and let it cool completely. Place the Alfredo sauce and beans in a skillet. Cook over low heat for 3-5 minutes. Stir in the rice to coat. Serve immediately

83) KOREAN-STYLE MILLET

Preparation Time: 30 minutes

Servings: 4

Ingredients:
- 1 cup dried millet, drained
- 1 tsp gochugaru flakes
- Salt and black pepper to taste

Directions:
- Place the millet and gochugaru flakes in a pot. Cover with enough water and bring to a boil. Lower the heat and simmer for 20 minutes. Drain and let cool. Transfer to a serving bowl and season with salt and pepper. Serve

84) LEMONY CHICKPEAS WITH KALE

Preparation Time: 20 minutes

Servings: 4

Ingredients:

- 4 tbsp olive oil
- 1 (15-oz) can chickpeas
- 1 onion, chopped
- 2 garlic cloves, minced
- 1 tbsp Italian seasoning
- 2 cups kale, chopped
- Sea salt and black pepper to taste
- Juice and zest of 1 lemon

Directions:

- Heat the oil in a skillet over medium heat. Place in chickpeas and cook for 5 minutes. Add in onion, garlic, Italian seasoning, and kale and cook for 5 minutes until the kale wilts. Stir in salt, lemon juice, lemon zest, and pepper. Serve warm

85) DINNER RICE AND LENTILS

Preparation Time: 25 minutes

Servings: 4

Ingredients:

- 2 tbsp olive oil
- 4 scallions, chopped
- 1 carrot, diced
- 1 celery stalk, chopped
- 2 (15-oz) cans lentils, drained
- 1 (15-oz) can diced tomatoes
- 1 tbsp dried rosemary
- 1 tsp ground coriander
- 1 tbsp garlic powder
- 2 cups cooked brown rice
- Sea salt and black pepper to taste

Directions:

- Heat the oil in a pot over medium heat. Place in scallions, carrot, and celery and cook for 5 minutes until tender. Stir in lentils, tomatoes, rosemary, coriander, and garlic powder. Lower the heat and simmer for 5-7 minutes. Mix in rice, salt, and pepper and cook another 2-3 minutes. Serve

86) SESAME KALE SLAW

Preparation Time: 15 minutes

Servings: 4

Ingredients:

- ¼ cup tahini
- 2 tbsp white miso paste
- 1 tbsp rice vinegar
- 1 tbsp toasted sesame oil
- 2 tsp soy sauce
- 1 (12-oz) bag kale slaw
- 2 scallions, minced
- ¼ cup toasted sesame seeds

Directions:

- In a bowl, combine the tahini, miso, vinegar, oil, and soy sauce. Stir in kale slaw, scallions, and sesame seeds. Let sit for 20 minutes. Serve immediately

87) SPICY STEAMED BROCCOLI

Preparation Time: 15 minutes

Servings: 6

Ingredients:

- 1 large head broccoli, into florets
- Salt to taste
- **1 tsp red pepper flakes**

Directions:

- Boil 1 cup water in a pot over medium heat. Place in a steamer basket and put in the florets. Steam covered for 5-7 minutes. In a bowl, toss the broccoli with red pepper flakes and salt. Serve

88) GARLIC ROASTED CARROTS

Preparation Time: 35 minutes

Servings: 4

Ingredients:

- 2 lb carrots, chopped into ¾ inch cubes
- 2 tsp olive oil
- ½ tsp chili powder
- ½ tsp smoked paprika
- ½ tsp dried oregano
- ½ tsp dried thyme
- ½ tsp garlic powder
- Salt to taste

Directions:

- Preheat oven to 400 F. Line with parchment paper a baking sheet. Rinse the carrots and pat dry. Chop into ¾ inch cubes. Place in a bowl and toss with olive oil.
- In a bowl, mix chili powder, paprika, oregano, thyme, olive oil, salt, and garlic powder. Pour over the carrots and toss to coat. Transfer to a greased baking sheet and bake for 30 minutes, turn once by half

89) EGGPLANT AND HUMMUS PIZZA

Preparation Time: 25 minutes

Servings: 2

Ingredients:

- ½ eggplant, sliced
- ½ red onion, sliced
- 1 cup cherry tomatoes, halved
- 3 tbsp chopped black olives
- Salt to taste
- Drizzle olive oil
- 2 prebaked pizza crusts
- ½ cup hummus
- 2 tbsp oregano

Directions:

- Preheat oven to 390 F,
- In a bowl, combine the eggplant, onion, tomatoes, olives, and salt. Toss to coat. Sprinkle with some olive oil. Arrange the crusts on a baking sheet and spread the hummus on each pizza. Top with the eggplant mixture. Bake for 20-30 minutes. Serve warm

90) MISO GREEN CABBAGE

Preparation Time: 50 minutes

Servings: 4

Ingredients:

- 1 lb green cabbage, halved
- 2 tsp olive
- 3 tsp miso paste
- 1 tsp dried oregano
- ½ tsp dried rosemary
- 1 tbsp balsamic vinegar

Directions:

- Preheat oven to 390 F. Line with parchment paper a baking sheet.
- Put the green cabbage in a bowl. Coat with olive oil, miso, oregano, rosemary, salt, and pepper. Remove to the baking sheet and bake for 35-40 minutes, shaking every 5 minutes until tender. Remove from the oven to a plate. Drizzle with balsamic vinegar and serve

91) STEAMED BROCCOLI WITH HAZELNUTS

Preparation Time: 20 minutes

Servings: 4

Ingredients:

- 1 lb broccoli, cut into florets
- 2 tbsp olive oil
- 3 garlic cloves, minced
- 1 cup sliced white mushrooms
- ¼ cup dry white wine
- 2 tbsp minced fresh parsley
- Salt and black pepper to taste
- ½ cup slivered toasted hazelnuts

Directions:

- Steam the broccoli for 8 minutes or until tender. Remove and set aside.
- Heat 1 tbsp of oil in a skillet over medium heat. Add in garlic and mushrooms and sauté for 5 minutes until tender. Pour in the wine and cook for 1 minute. Stir in broccoli, parsley, salt, and pepper. Cook for 3 minutes, until the liquid has reduced. Remove to a bowl and add in the remaining oil and hazelnuts and toss to coat. Serve warm

92) CILANTRO OKRA

Preparation Time: 10 minutes

Servings: 4

Ingredients:

- 2 tbsp olive oil
- 4 cups okra, halved
- Sea salt and black pepper to taste
- 3 tbsp chopped fresh cilantro

Directions:

- Heat the oil in a skillet over medium heat. Place in the okra, cook for 5 minutes. Turn the heat off and mix in salt, pepper, and cilantro. Serve immediately

93) CITRUS ASPARAGUS

Preparation Time: 15 minutes

Servings: 4

Ingredients:

- 1 onion, minced
- 2 tsp lemon zest
- 1/3 cup fresh lemon juice
- 1 tbsp olive oil
- Salt and black pepper to taste
- 1 lb asparagus, trimmed

Directions:

- Combine the onion, lemon zest, lemon juice, and oil in a bowl. Sprinkle with salt and pepper. Let sit for 5-10 minutes.
- Insert a steamer basket and 1 cup of water in a pot over medium heat. Place the asparagus on the basket and steam for 4-5 minutes until tender but crispy. Leave to cool for 10 minutes, then arrange on a plate. Serve drizzled with the dressing

The Plant-Based for Athlete

Snacks

SNACKS

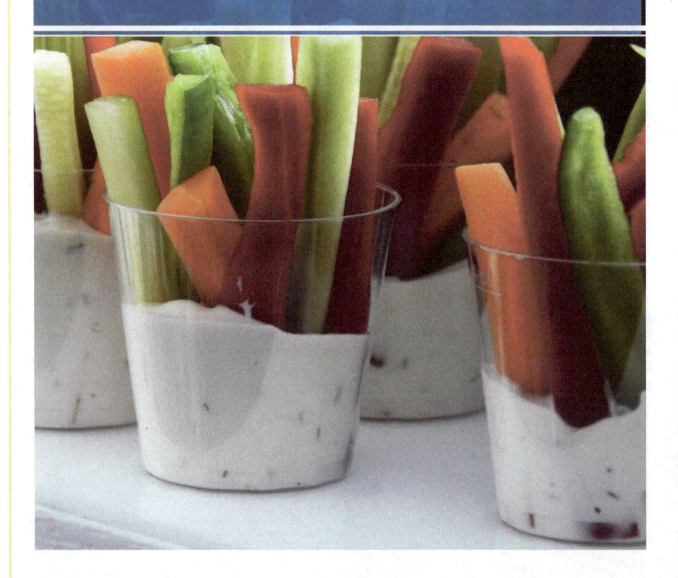

The Plant-Based for Athlete

94) SESAME CABBAGE SAUTÉ

Preparation Time: 15 minutes

Servings: 4

Ingredients:

- 2 tbsp soy sauce
- 1 tbsp toasted sesame oil
- 1 tbsp hot sauce
- ½ tbsp pure date sugar
- ½ tbsp olive oil
- 1 head green cabbage, shredded
- 2 carrots, julienned
- 3 green onions, thinly sliced
- 2 garlic cloves, minced
- 1 tbsp fresh grated ginger
- Salt and black pepper to taste
- 1 tbsp sesame seeds

Directions:

- In a small bowl, mix the soy sauce, sesame oil, hot sauce, and date sugar.
- Heat the olive oil in a large skillet and sauté the cabbage, carrots, green onion, garlic, and ginger until softened, 5 minutes. Mix in the prepared sauce and toss well. Cook for 1 to 2 minutes. Dish the food and garnish with the sesame seeds

95) TOMATOES STUFFED WITH CHICKPEAS AND QUINOA

Preparation Time: 50 minutes

Servings: 4

Ingredients:

- 8 medium tomatoes
- ¾ cup quinoa, rinsed and drained
- 1 ½ cups water
- 1 tbsp olive oil
- 1 small onion, diced
- 3 garlic cloves, minced
- 1 cup chopped spinach
- 1 (7 oz) can chickpeas, drained
- ½ cup chopped fresh basil

Directions:

- Preheat the oven to 400 F.
- Cut off the heads of tomatoes and use a paring knife to scoop the inner pulp of the tomatoes. Season with some olive oil, salt, and black pepper. Add the quinoa and water to a medium pot, season with salt, and cook until the quinoa is tender and the water absorbs, 10 to 15 minutes. Fluff and set aside.
- Heat the remaining olive oil in a skillet and sauté the onion and garlic for 30 seconds. Mix in the spinach and cook until wilted, 2 minutes. Stir in the basil, chickpeas, and quinoa; allow warming from 2 minutes.
- Spoon the mixture into the tomatoes, place the tomatoes into the baking dish and bake in the oven for 20 minutes or until the tomatoes soften. Remove the tomatoes from the oven and dish the food

96) HERBED VEGETABLE TRAYBAKE

Preparation Time: 85 minutes

Servings: 4

Ingredients:

- 2 tbsp plant butter
- 1 large onion, diced
- 1 cup celery, diced
- ½ cup carrots, diced
- ½ tsp dried marjoram
- 2 cups chopped cremini mushrooms
- 1 cup vegetable broth
- ¼ cup chopped fresh parsley
- 1 whole-grain bread loaf, cubed

Directions:

- Melt the butter in a large skillet and sauté onion, celery, mushrooms, and carrots for 5 minutes. Mix in marjoram, salt, and pepper. Pour in the vegetable broth and mix in parsley and bread. Cook until the broth reduces by half, 10 minutes. Pour the mixture into a baking dish and cover with foil. Bake in the oven at 375 F for 30 minutes. Uncover and bake further for 30 minutes or until golden brown on top, and the liquid absorbs. Remove the dish from the oven and serve the stuffing

97) LOUISIANA-STYLE SWEET POTATO CHIPS

Preparation Time: 55 minutes

Servings: 4

Ingredients:

- 2 sweet potatoes, peeled and sliced
- 2 tbsp melted plant butter
- 1 tbsp Cajun seasoning

Directions:

- Preheat the oven to 400 F and line a baking sheet with parchment paper.
- In a medium bowl, add the sweet potatoes, salt, plant butter, and Cajun seasoning. Toss well. Spread the chips on the baking sheet, making sure not to overlap, and bake in the oven for 50 minutes to 1 hour or until crispy. Remove the sheet and pour the chips into a large bowl. Allow cooling and enjoy

98) BELL PEPPER AND SEITAN BALLS

Preparation Time: 25 minutes

Servings: 4

Ingredients:

- 1 tbsp flaxseed powder
- 1 lb seitan, crumbled
- ¼ cup chopped mixed bell peppers
- Salt and black pepper to taste
- 1 tbsp almond flour
- 1 tsp garlic powder
- 1 tsp onion powder
- 1 tsp tofu mayonnaise
- Olive oil for brushing

Directions:

- Preheat the oven to 400 F and line a baking sheet with parchment paper.
- In a bowl, mix flaxseed powder with 3 tbsp water and allow thickening for 5 minutes. Add in seitan, bell peppers, salt, pepper, almond flour, garlic powder, onion powder, and tofu mayonnaise. Mix and form 1-inch balls from the mixture. Arrange on the baking sheet, brush with cooking spray, and bake in the oven for 15 to 20 minutes or until brown and compacted. Remove from the oven and serve

99) PARMESAN BROCCOLI TOTS

Preparation Time: 30 minutes

Servings: 4

Ingredients:

- 1 tbsp flaxseed powder
- 1 head broccoli, cut into florets
- 2/3 cup toasted almond flour
- 2 garlic cloves, minced
- 2 cups grated plant-based Parmesan
- Salt to taste

Directions:

- Preheat the oven to 350 F and line a baking sheet with parchment paper.
- In a small bowl, mix the flaxseed powder with the 3 tbsp water and allow thickening for 5 minutes to make the vegan "flax egg". Place the broccoli in a safe microwave bowl, sprinkle with 2 tbsp of water, and steam in the microwave for 1 minute or until softened. Transfer the broccoli to a food processor and add the vegan "flax egg," almond flour, garlic, plant cheese, and salt. Blend until coarsely smooth.
- Pour the mixture into a bowl and form 2-inch oblong balls from the mixture. Place the tots on the baking sheet and bake in the oven for 15 to 20 minutes or until firm and compacted. Remove the tots from the oven and serve warm with tomato dipping sauce.

100) CHOCOLATE BARS WITH WALNUTS

Preparation Time: 60 minutes

Servings: 4

Ingredients:

- 1 cup walnuts
- 3 tbsp sunflower seeds
- 2 tbsp unsweetened chocolate chips
- 1 tbsp unsweetened cocoa powder
- 1 ½ tsp vanilla extract
- ¼ tsp cinnamon powder
- 2 tbsp melted coconut oil
- 2 tbsp toasted almond meal
- 2 tsp pure maple syrup

Directions:

- In a food processor, add the walnuts, sunflower seeds, chocolate chips, cocoa powder, vanilla extract, cinnamon powder, coconut oil, almond meal, maple syrup, and blitz a few times until combined.
- Line a flat baking sheet with plastic wrap, pour the mixture onto the sheet and place another plastic wrap on top. Use a rolling pin to flatten the batter and then remove the top plastic wrap. Freeze the snack until firm, 1 hour. Remove from the freezer, cut into 1 ½-inch sized bars and enjoy immediately

101) CARROT ENERGY BALLS

Preparation Time: 10 minutes + chilling time

Servings: 8

Ingredients:

- 1 large carrot, grated carrot
- 1 ½ cups old-fashioned oats
- 1 cup raisins
- 1 cup dates, pitied
- 1 cup coconut flakes
- 1/4 tsp ground cloves
- 1/2 tsp ground cinnamon

Directions:

- In your food processor, pulse all ingredients until it forms a sticky and uniform mixture.
- Shape the batter into equal balls.
- Place in your refrigerator until ready to serve. Enjoy

102) CRUNCHY SWEET POTATO BITES

Preparation Time: 25 minutes + chilling time

Servings: 4

Ingredients:
- 4 sweet potatoes, peeled and grated
- 2 chia eggs
- 1/4 cup nutritional yeast
- 2 tbsp tahini
- 2 tbsp chickpea flour
- 1 tsp shallot powder
- 1 tsp garlic powder
- 1 tsp paprika
- Sea salt and ground black pepper, to taste

Directions:
- Start by preheating your oven to 395 degrees F. Line a baking pan with parchment paper or Silpat mat.
- Thoroughly combine all the ingredients until everything is well incorporated.
- Roll the batter into equal balls and place them in your refrigerator for about 1 hour.
- Bake these balls for approximately 25 minutes, turning them over halfway through the cooking time. Enjoy

103) ROASTED GLAZED BABY CARROTS

Preparation Time: 30 minutes

Servings: 6

Ingredients:
- 2 pounds baby carrots
- 1/4 cup olive oil
- 1/4 cup apple cider vinegar
- 1/2 tsp red pepper flakes
- Sea salt and freshly ground black pepper, to taste
- 1 tbsp agave syrup
- 2 tbsp soy sauce
- 1 tbsp fresh cilantro, minced

Directions:
- Start by preheating your oven 395 degrees F.
- Then, toss the carrots with the olive oil, vinegar, red pepper, salt, black pepper, agave syrup and soy sauce.
- Roast the carrots for about 30 minutes, rotating the pan once or twice. Garnish with fresh cilantro and serve. Enjoy

104) OVEN-BAKED KALE CHIPS

Preparation Time: 20 minutes

Servings: 8

Ingredients:
- 2 bunches kale, leaves separated
- 2 tbsp olive oil
- 1/2 tsp mustard seeds
- 1/2 tsp celery seeds
- 1/2 tsp dried oregano
- 1/4 tsp ground cumin
- 1 tsp garlic powder
- Coarse sea salt and ground black pepper, to taste

Directions:
- Start by preheating your oven to 340 degrees F. Line a baking sheet with parchment paper or Silpat mar.
- Toss the kale leaves with the remaining ingredients until well coated.
- Bake in the preheated oven for about 13 minutes, rotating the pan once or twice. Enjoy

105) CHEESY CASHEW DIP

Preparation Time: 10 minutes

Servings: 8

Ingredients:
- 1 cup raw cashews
- 1 lemon, freshly squeezed
- 2 tbsp tahini
- 2 tbsp nutritional yeast
- 1/2 tsp turmeric powder
- 1/2 tsp red pepper flakes, crushed
- Sea salt and ground black pepper, to taste

Directions:
- Place all the ingredients in the bowl of your food processor. Blend until uniform, creamy and smooth. You can add a splash of water to thin it out, as needed.
- Spoon your dip into a serving bowl; serve with veggie sticks, chips, or crackers.
- Enjoy

106) PEPPERY HUMMUS DIP

Preparation Time: 10 minutes

Servings: 10

Ingredients:

- 20 ounces canned or boiled chickpeas, drained
- 1/4 cup tahini
- 2 garlic cloves, minced
- 2 tbsp lemon juice, freshly squeezed
- 1/2 cup chickpea liquid
- 2 red roasted peppers, seeded and sliced
- 1/2 tsp paprika
- 1 tsp dried basil
- Sea salt and ground black pepper, to taste
- 2 tbsp olive oil

Directions:

- Blitz all the ingredients, except for the oil, in your blender or food processor until your desired consistency is reached.
- Place in your refrigerator until ready to serve.
- Serve with toasted pita wedges or chips, if desired. Enjoy

107) TRADITIONAL LEBANESE MUTABAL

Preparation Time: 10 minutes

Servings: 6

Ingredients:

- 1 pound eggplant
- 1 onion, chopped
- 1 tbsp garlic paste
- 4 tbsp tahini
- 1 tbsp coconut oil
- 2 tbsp lemon juice
- 1/2 tsp ground coriander
- 1/4 cup ground cloves
- 1 tsp red pepper flakes
- 1 tsp smoked peppers
- Sea salt and ground black pepper, to taste

Directions:

- Roast the eggplant until the skin turns black; peel the eggplant and transfer it to the bowl of your food processor.
- Add in the remaining ingredients. Blend until everything is well incorporated.
- Serve with crostini or pita bread, if desired. Enjoy

108) INDIAN-STYLE ROASTED CHICKPEAS

Preparation Time: 10 minutes

Servings: 8

Ingredients:

- 2 cups canned chickpeas, drained
- 2 tbsp olive oil
- 1/2 tsp garlic powder
- 1/2 tsp paprika
- 1 tsp curry powder
- 1 tsp garam masala
- Sea salt and red pepper, to taste

Directions:

- Pat the chickpeas dry using paper towels. Drizzle olive oil over the chickpeas.
- Roast the chickpeas in the preheated oven at 400 degrees F for about 25 minutes, tossing them once or twice.
- Toss your chickpeas with the spices and enjoy

109) AVOCADO WITH TAHINI SAUCE

Preparation Time: 10 minutes

Servings: 4

Ingredients:

- 2 large-sized avocados, pitted and halved
- 4 tbsp tahini
- 4 tbsp soy sauce
- 1 tbsp lemon juice
- 1/2 tsp red pepper flakes
- Sea salt and ground black pepper, to taste
- 1 tsp garlic powder

Directions:

- Place the avocado halves on a serving platter.
- Mix the tahini, soy sauce, lemon juice, red pepper, salt, black pepper and garlic powder in a small bowl. Divide the sauce between the avocado halves.
- Enjoy

Desserts

The Plant-Based for Athlete

DESSERTS

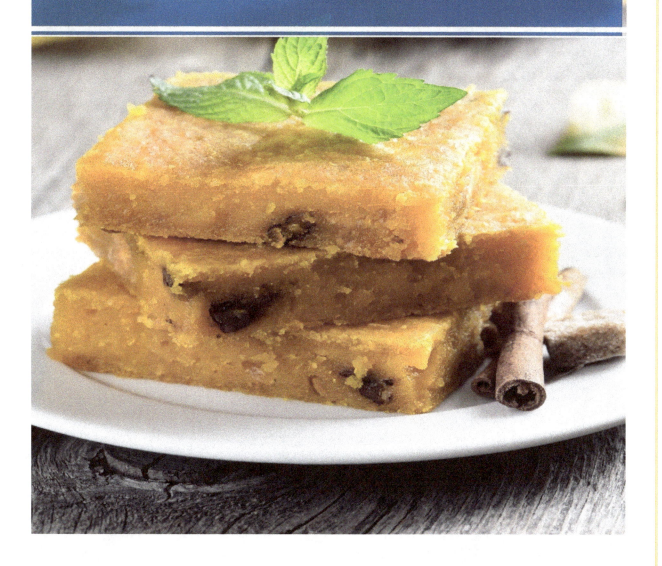

110) CHOCOLATE DREAM BALLS

Preparation Time: 10 minutes + chilling time

Servings: 8

Ingredients:

- 3 tbsp cocoa powder
- 8 fresh dates, pitted and soaked for 15 minutes
- 2 tbsp tahini, at room temperature
- 1/2 tsp ground cinnamon
- 1/2 cup vegan chocolate, broken into chunks
- 1 tbsp coconut oil, at room temperature

Directions:

- Add the cocoa powder, dates, tahini and cinnamon to the bowl of your food processor. Process until the mixture forms a ball.
- Use a cookie scoop to portion the mixture into 1-ounce portions. Roll the balls and refrigerate them for at least 30 minutes.
- Meanwhile, microwave the chocolate until melted; add in the coconut oil and whisk to combine well.
- Dip the chocolate balls in the coating and store them in your refrigerator until ready to serve. Enjoy

111) LAST-MINUTE MACAROONS

Preparation Time: 15 minutes

Servings: 10

Ingredients:

- 3 cups coconut flakes, sweetened
- 9 ounces canned coconut milk, sweetened
- 1 tsp ground anise
- 1 tsp vanilla extract

Directions:

- Begin by preheating your oven to 325 degrees F. Line the cookie sheets with parchment paper.
- Thoroughly combine all the ingredients until everything is well incorporated.
- Use a cookie scoop to drop mounds of the batter onto the prepared cookie sheets.
- Bake for about 11 minutes until they are lightly browned. Enjoy

112)

113) OLD-FASHIONED RATAFIAS

Preparation Time: 20 minutes

Servings: 8

Ingredients:

- 2 ounces all-purpose flour
- 2 ounces almond flour
- 1 tsp baking powder
- 2 tbsp applesauce
- 5 ounces caster sugar
- 1 ½ ounces vegan butter
- 4 drops of ratafia essence

Directions:

- Start by preheating your oven to 330 degrees F. Line a cookie sheet with parchment paper.
- Thoroughly combine all the ingredients until everything is well incorporated.
- Use a cookie scoop to drop mounds of the batter onto the prepared cookie sheet.
- Bake for about 15 minutes until they are lightly browned. Enjoy

114) JASMINE RICE PUDDING WITH DRIED APRICOTS

Preparation Time: 20 minutes

Servings: 4

Ingredients:

- 1 cup jasmine rice, rinsed
- 1 cup water
- 1 cup almond milk
- 1/2 cup brown sugar
- A pinch of salt
- A pinch of grated nutmeg
- 1/2 cup dried apricots, chopped
- 1/4 tsp cinnamon powder
- 1 tsp vanilla extract

Directions:

- Add the rice and water to a saucepan. Cover the saucepan and bring the water to a boil.
- Turn the heat to low; let it simmer for another 10 minutes until all the water is absorbed.
- Then, add in the remaining ingredients and stir to combine. Let it simmer for 10 minutes more or until the pudding has thickened. Enjoy

115) CHOCOLATE FUDGE WITH NUTS

Preparation Time: 10 minutes + cooling time

Servings: 4

Ingredients:

- 3 cups chocolate chips
- ¼ cup thick coconut milk
- 1 ½ tsp vanilla extract
- A pinch salt
- 1 cup chopped mixed nuts

Directions:

- Line a square pan with baking paper. Melt the chocolate chips, coconut milk, and vanilla in a medium pot over low heat. Mix in the salt and nuts until well distributed and pour the mixture into the square pan. Refrigerate for at least 2 hours. Remove from the fridge, cut into squares, and serve

116) CHOCOLATE AND PEANUT BUTTER COOKIES

Preparation Time: 15 minutes + cooling time

Servings: 4

Ingredients:

- 1 tbsp flaxseed powder
- 1 cup pure date sugar + for dusting
- ½ cup vega butter, softened
- ½ cup creamy peanut butter
- 1 tsp vanilla extract
- 1 ¾ cup whole-wheat flour
- 1 tsp baking soda
- ¼ tsp salt
- ¼ cup unsweetened chocolate chips

Directions:

- In a small bowl, mix the flaxseed powder with 3 tbsp water and allow thickening for 5 minutes to make the vegan "flax egg." In a medium bowl, whisk the date sugar, plant butter, and peanut butter until light and fluffy. Mix in the flax egg and vanilla until combined. Add in flour, baking soda, salt, and whisk well again. Fold in chocolate chips, cover the bowl with plastic wrap, and refrigerate for 1 hour.
- Preheat oven to 375 F and line a baking sheet with parchment paper. Use a cookie sheet to scoop mounds of the batter onto the sheet with 1-inch intervals. Bake for 10 minutes. Remove the cookies from the oven, cool for 3 minutes, roll in some date sugar, and serve

117) MIXED BERRY YOGURT ICE POPS

Preparation Time: 5 minutes + chilling time

Servings: 6

Ingredients:

- 2/3 cup avocado, halved and pitted
- 2/3 cup frozen berries, thawed
- 1 cup dairy-free yogurt
- ½ cup coconut cream
- 1 tsp vanilla extract

Directions:

- Pour the avocado pulp, berries, dairy-free yogurt, coconut cream, and vanilla extract. Process until smooth. Pour into ice pop sleeves and freeze for 8 or more hours. Enjoy the ice pops when ready

118) HOLIDAY PECAN TART

Preparation Time: 50 minutes + cooling time

Servings: 4

Ingredients:

- 4 tbsp flaxseed powder
- 1/3 cup whole-wheat flour
- ½ tsp salt
- ¼ cup cold plant butter, crumbled
- 3 tbsp pure malt syrup
- For the filling:
- 3 tbsp flaxseed powder + 9 tbsp water
- 2 cups toasted pecans, chopped
- 1 cup light corn syrup
- ½ cup pure date sugar
- 1 tbsp pure pomegranate molasses
- 4 tbsp plant butter, melted
- ½ tsp salt
- 2 tsp vanilla extract

Directions:

- Preheat oven to 350 F. In a bowl, mix the flaxseed powder with 12 tbsp water and allow thickening for 5 minutes. Do this for the filling's vegan "flax egg" too in a separate bowl. In a bowl, combine flour and salt. Add in plant butter and whisk until crumbly. Pour in the crust's vegan "flax egg" and maple syrup and mix until smooth dough forms. Flatten the dough on a flat surface, cover with plastic wrap, and refrigerate for 1 hour. Dust a working surface with flour, remove the dough onto the surface, and using a rolling pin, flatten the dough into a 1-inch diameter circle. Lay the dough on a greased pie pan and press to fit the shape of the pan. Trim the edges of the pan. Lay a parchment paper on the dough, pour on some baking beans and bake for 20 minutes. Remove, pour out baking beans, and allow cooling.
- In a bowl, mix the filling's vegan "flax egg," pecans, corn syrup, date sugar, pomegranate molasses, plant butter, salt, and vanilla. Pour and spread the mixture on the piecrust. Bake for 20 minutes or until the filling sets. Remove from the oven, decorate with more pecans, slice, and cool. Slice and serve

119) COCONUT CHOCOLATE BARKS

Preparation Time: 35 minutes

Servings: 4

Ingredients:

- 1/3 cup coconut oil, melted
- ¼ cup almond butter, melted
- 2 tbsp unsweetened coconut flakes.
- 1 tsp pure maple syrup
- A pinch of ground rock salt
- ¼ cup unsweetened cocoa nibs

Directions:

- Line a baking tray with baking paper and set aside. In a medium bowl, mix the coconut oil, almond butter, coconut flakes, maple syrup, and fold in the rock salt and cocoa nibs. Pour and spread the mixture on the baking sheet, chill in the refrigerator for 20 minutes or until firm. Remove the dessert, break into shards, and enjoy. Preserve extras in the refrigerator

120) NUTTY DATE CAKE

Preparation Time: 1 hour 30 minutes

Servings: 4

Ingredients:

- ½ cup cold plant butter, cut into pieces
- 1 tbsp flaxseed powder
- ½ cup whole-wheat flour
- ¼ cup chopped pecans and walnuts
- 1 tsp baking powder
- 1 tsp baking soda
- 1 tsp cinnamon powder
- 1 tsp salt
- 1/3 cup pitted dates, chopped
- ½ cup pure date sugar
- 1 tsp vanilla extract
- ¼ cup pure date syrup for drizzling

Directions:

- Preheat oven to 350 F and lightly grease a baking dish with some plant butter. In a small bowl, mix the flaxseed powder with 3 tbsp water and allow thickening for 5 minutes to make the vegan "flax egg."
- In a food processor, add the flour, nuts, baking powder, baking soda, cinnamon powder, and salt. Blend until well combined. Add 1/3 cup of water, dates, date sugar, and vanilla. Process until smooth with tiny pieces of dates evident.
- Pour the batter into the baking dish and bake in the oven for 1 hour and 10 minutes or until a toothpick inserted comes out clean. Remove the dish from the oven, invert the cake onto a serving platter to cool, drizzle with the date syrup, slice, and serve

121) BERRY CUPCAKES WITH CASHEW CHEESE ICING

Preparation Time: 35 minutes + cooling time

Servings: 4

Ingredients:

- 2 cups whole-wheat flour
- ¼ cup corn-starch
- 2 ½ tsp baking powder
- 1 ½ cups pure date sugar
- ½ tsp salt
- ¾ cup plant butter, softened
- 3 tsp vanilla extract
- 1 cup strawberries, pureed
- 1 cup oat milk, room temperature
- ¾ cup cashew cream
- 2 tbsp coconut oil, melted
- 3 tbsp pure maple syrup
- 1 tsp vanilla extract
- 1 tsp freshly squeezed lemon juice

Directions:

- Preheat the oven to 350 F and line a 12-holed muffin tray with cupcake liners. Set aside.
- In a bowl, mix flour, corn-starch, baking powder, date sugar, and salt. Whisk in plant butter, vanilla extract, strawberries, and oat milk until well combined. Divide the mixture into the muffin cups two-thirds way up and bake for 20-25 minutes. Allow cooling while you make the frosting.
- In a blender, add cashew cream, coconut oil, maple syrup, vanilla, and lemon juice. Process until smooth. Pour the frosting into a medium bowl and chill for 30 minutes. Transfer the mixture into a piping bag and swirl mounds of the frosting onto the cupcakes. Serve immediately

122) COCONUT AND CHOCOLATE CAKE

Preparation Time: 40 minutes + cooling time

Servings: 4

Ingredients:

- 2/3 cup toasted almond flour
- ¼ cup unsalted plant butter, melted
- 2 cups chocolate bars, cubed
- 2 ½ cups coconut cream
- Fresh berries for topping

Directions:

- Lightly grease a 9-inch springform pan with some plant butter and set aside.
- Mix the almond flour and plant butter in a medium bowl and pour the mixture into the springform pan. Use the spoon to spread and press the mixture into the bottom of the pan. Place in the refrigerator to firm for 30 minutes.
- Meanwhile, pour the chocolate in a safe microwave bowl and melt for 1 minute stirring every 30 seconds. Remove from the microwave and mix in the coconut cream and maple syrup.
- Remove the cake pan from the oven, pour the chocolate mixture on

top, and shake the pan and even the layer. Chill further for 4 to 6 hours. Take out the pan from the fridge, release the cake and garnish with the raspberries or strawberries. Slice and serve

123) BERRY MACEDONIA WITH MINT

Preparation Time: 20 minutes

Servings: 4

Ingredients:

- ¼ cup lemon juice
- 4 tsp agave syrup
- 2 cups chopped pears
- 2 cups chopped strawberries
- 3 cups mixed berries
- 8 fresh mint leaves

Directions:

- Chop half of the mint leaves; reserve.
- In a large bowl, combine together pears, strawberries, raspberries, blackberries, and half of the mint leaves. Divide the Macedonia salad between 4 small cups. Top with lemon juice, agave syrup, and mint leaves and serve chilled

124) CINNAMON PUMPKIN PIE

Preparation Time: 1 hr 10 min + cooling time

Servings: 4

Ingredients:

- For the piecrust:
- 4 tbsp flaxseed powder
- 1/3 cup whole-wheat flour
- ½ tsp salt
- ¼ cup cold plant butter, crumbled
- 3 tbsp pure malt syrup
- For the filling:
- 2 tbsp flaxseed powder + 6 tbsp water
- 4 tbsp plant butter
- ¼ cup pure maple syrup
- ¼ cup pure date sugar
- 1 tsp cinnamon powder
- ½ tsp ginger powder
- 1/8 tsp cloves powder
- 1 (15 oz) can pumpkin purée
- 1 cup almond milk

Directions:

- Preheat oven to 350 F. In a bowl, mix flaxseed powder with 12 tbsp water and allow thickening for 5 minutes. Do this for the filling's vegan "flax egg" too in another bowl. In a bowl, combine flour and salt. Add in plant butter and whisk until crumbly. Pour in crust's vegan "flax egg," maple syrup, vanilla, and mix until smooth dough forms. Flatten, cover with plastic wrap, and refrigerate for 1 hour.
- Dust a working surface with flour, remove the dough onto the surface and flatten it into a 1-inch diameter circle. Lay the dough on a greased pie pan and press to fit the shape of the pan. Use a knife to trim the edges of the pan. Lay a parchment paper on the dough, pour on some baking beans and bake for 15-20 minutes. Remove, pour out the baking beans, and allow cooling. In a bowl, whisk filling's flaxseed, butter, maple syrup, date sugar, cinnamon powder, ginger powder, cloves powder, pumpkin puree, and almond milk. Pour the mixture onto the piecrust and bake for 35-40 minutes

125) PARTY MATCHA AND HAZELNUT CHEESECAKE

Preparation Time: 20 minutes + cooling time

Servings: 4

Ingredients:

- 2/3 cup toasted rolled oats
- ¼ cup plant butter, melted
- 3 tbsp pure date sugar
- 6 oz cashew cream cheese
- ¼ cup almond milk
- 1 tbsp matcha powder
- ¼ cup just-boiled water
- 3 tsp agar agar powder
- 2 tbsp toasted hazelnuts, chopped

Directions:

- Process the oats, butter, and date sugar in a blender until smooth.
- Pour the mixture into a greased 9-inch springform pan and press the mixture onto the bottom of the pan. Refrigerate for 30 minutes until firm while you make the filling.
- In a large bowl, using an electric mixer, whisk the cashew cream cheese until smooth. Beat in the almond milk and mix in the matcha powder until smooth.
- Mix the boiled water and agar agar until dissolved and whisk this mixture into the creamy mix. Fold in the hazelnuts until well distributed. Remove the cake pan from the fridge and pour in the cream mixture. Shake the pan to ensure a smooth layering on top. Refrigerate further for at least 3 hours. Take out the cake pan, release the cake, slice, and serve

THE PLANT-BASED DIET
FOR ONE

The Revolutionary Recipe Book with Easy and Tasty Recipes for Healthy Lifestyle and Smart People!

Lose Rapidly Weight with a Large Choice of 120+ Vegan and Vegetarian Recipes!

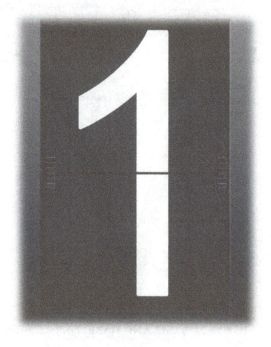

By

Audrey Pottery

TABLE OF CONTENT

The Plant-Based for Athlete

INTRODUCTION to PLANT-BASED DIET 69

FOOD TO AVOID 71

BREAKFAST 73

    1) Banana Pancakes 74

    2) Pesto Bread 74

    3) Classic French Toasts 74

    4) Creamy Bread with Sesame 75

    5) Different Seeds Bread 75

    6) Naan Bread 76

    7) Mushroom and Spinach Chickpea Omelette 76

    8) Coconut-Raspberry Pancakes 77

    9) Blueberry-Chia Pudding 77

    10) Potato and Cauliflower Browns 78

    11) Pistachios-Pumpkin Cake 79

    12) Bell Pepper with Scrambled Tofu 79

    13) Original French Toast 80

    14) Frybread with Peanut Butter and Jam 80

    15) Pudding with Sultanas on Ciabatta Bread 81

    16) Vegan Banh Mi 81

    17) Breakfast Nutty Oatmeal Muffins 81

    18) Smoothie Bowl of Raspberry and Chia 82

    19) Breakfast Oats with Walnuts and Currants 82

    20) Applesauce Pancakes with Coconut 82

    21) Veggie Panini 83

    22) Cheddar Grits and Soy Chorizo 84

    23) Vanilla Crepes and Berry Cream Compote Topping 84

24) Strawberry and Pecan Breakfast 85
25) Granola with Hazelnuts and Orange 85
26) Orange Crepes 86
27) Oat Bread with Coconut 86
28) Bowl with Black Beans and Spicy Quinoa 86
29) Almond and Raisin Granola 87
30) Pecan and Pumpkin Seed Oat Jars 87
31) Easy Apple Muffins 87
32) Almond Yogurt with Berries and Walnuts 88
33) Breakfast Blueberry Muesli 88
34) Berry and Almond Butter Swirl Bowl 89
35) Oats with Coconut and Strawberries 89

SOUPS, STEW, AND SALADS 90

36) Black Bean Quinoa Salad 91
37) Power Bulgur Salad with Herbs 91
38) ORIGINAL ROASTED Pepper Salad 92
39) Winter Hearty Quinoa Soup 92
40) Green Lentil Salad 93
41) Chickpea, Acorn Squash, and Couscous Soup 93
42) Garlic Crostini with Cabbage Soup 94
43) Green Bean Soup Cream 94
44) French Traditional Onion Soup 95
45) Roasted Carrot Soup 95
46) Italian Penne Pasta Salad 96
47) Chana Chaat Indian Salad 96
48) Tempeh and Noodle Salad Thai-Style 97

49)	Typical Cream of Broccoli Soup	97
50)	Raisin Moroccan Lentil Salad	98
51)	Chickpea and Asparagus Salad	98
52)	Quinoa and Avocado Salad	99
53)	Tabbouleh Salad with Tofu	99
54)	Green Pasta Salad	100
55)	Original Ukrainian Borscht	101
56)	Lentil Beluga Salad	101
57)	Indian Naan Salad	102
58)	Broccoli Ginger Soup	102
59)	Noodle Rice Soup with Beans	102
60)	Vegetable and Rice Soup	103
61)	Daikon and Sweet Potato Soup	103
62)	Chickpea and Vegetable Soup	103
63)	Italian-style Bean Soup	105
64)	Brussels Sprouts and Tofu Soup	105
65)	White Bean Rosemary Soup	105
66)	Mushroom and Tofu Soup	106
67)	Autumn Root Vegetable Soup	106
68)	Greek Salad	106

VEGETABLES AND SIDE DISHES 108

69)	Chinese Cabbage Stir-Fry	109
70)	Sautéed Cauliflower with Sesame Seeds	109
71)	Sweet Mashed Carrots	110
72)	Sautéed Turnip Greens	110
73)	Yukon Gold Mashed Potatoes	111

74)	Aromatic Sautéed Swiss Chard	111
75)	Classic Sautéed Bell Peppers	111
76)	Mashed Root Vegetables	112
77)	Roasted Butternut Squash	112
78)	Sautéed Cremini Mushrooms	112
79)	Roasted Asparagus with Sesame Seeds	113
80)	Greek-Style Eggplant Skillet	113
81)	Cauliflower Rice	114
82)	Garlicky Kale	114
83)	Artichokes Braised in Lemon and Olive Oil	115
84)	Rosemary and Garlic Roasted Carrots	115

LUNCH 116

85)	Millet Porridge with Sultanas	117
86)	Quinoa Porridge with Dried Figs	117
87)	Bread Pudding with Raisins	117
88)	Bulgur Wheat Salad	118
89)	Rye Porridge with Blueberry Topping	118
90)	Coconut Sorghum Porridge	118
91)	Mum's Aromatic Rice	119
92)	Everyday Savory Grits	119
93)	Greek-Style Barley Salad	119
94)	Sweet Maize Meal Porridge	120
95)	Dad's Millet Muffins	120
96)	Ginger Brown Rice	120
97)	Chili Bean and Brown Rice Tortillas	121
98)	Cashew Buttered Quesadillas with Leafy Greens	122

99)	Asparagus with Creamy Puree	122
100)	Kale Mushroom Galette	123
101)	Focaccia with Mixed Mushrooms	124
102)	Seitan Cakes with Broccoli Mash	124
103)	Spicy Cheese with Tofu Balls	125
104)	Quinoa andVeggie Burgers	125
105)	Baked Tofu with Roasted Peppers	126
106)	Zoodle Bolognese	126
107)	Zucchini Boats with Vegan Cheese	127
108)	Roasted Butternut Squash with Chimichurri	127
109)	Sweet and Spicy Brussel Sprout Stir-Fry	128
110)	Black Bean Burgers with BBQ Sauce	128
111)	Creamy Brussels Sprouts Bake	129
112)	Basil Pesto Seitan Panini	129
113)	Sweet Oatmeal "Grits"	130
114)	Freekeh Bowl with Dried Figs	130
115)	Cornmeal Porridge with Maple Syrup	130

DINNER 131

116)	Matcha-Infused Tofu Rice	132
117)	Chinese Fried Rice	132
118)	Savory Seitan xand Bell Pepper Rice	133
119)	Asparagus and Mushrooms with Mashed Potatoes	133
120)	Green Pea and Lemon Couscous	133
121)	Chimichurri Fusili with Navy Beans	134
122)	Quinoa and Chickpea Pot	134
123)	Buckwheat Pilaf with Pine Nuts	135

124)	 135
125)	Italian Holiday Stuffing 135
126)	Pressure Cooker Green Lentils 135
127)	Cherry and Pistachio Bulgur 136
128)	Mushroom Fried Rice 136
129)	Bean and Brown Rice with Artichokes 136
130)	Pressure Cooker Celery and Spinach Chickpeas 137
131)	Veggie Paella with Lentils 137
132)	Curry Bean with Artichokes 138
133)	Endive Slaw with Olives 138
134)	Paprika Cauliflower Tacos 138

SNACKS 139

135)	Freekeh Salad with Za'atar 140
136)	Vegetable Amaranth Soup 140
137)	Polenta with Mushrooms and Chickpeas 141
138)	Teff Salad with Avocado and Beans 141
139)	Overnight Oatmeal with Walnuts 142
140)	Colorful Spelt Salad 142
141)	Powerful Teff Bowl with Tahini Sauce 143
142)	Polenta Toasts with Balsamic Onions 143
143)	Freekeh Pilaf with Chickpeas 144
144)	Grandma's Pilau with Garden Vegetables 144
145)	Easy Barley Risotto 145
146)	Traditional Portuguese Papas 145
147)	The Best Millet Patties Ever 145

DESSERTS 146

148)	Avocado Truffles with Chocolate Coating	147
149)	Vanilla Berry Tarts	147
150)	Homemade Chocolates with Coconut and Raisins	148
151)	Mocha Fudge	148
152)	Almond and Chocolate Chip Bars	148
153)	Almond Butter Cookies	149
154)	Peanut Butter Oatmeal Bars	149
155)	Vanilla Halvah Fudge	150
156)	Raw Chocolate Mango Pie	150
157)	Chocolate N'ice Cream	150
158)	Raw Raspberry Cheesecake	151
159)	Mini Lemon Tarts	151
160)	Coconut Blondies with Raisins	152
161)	Chocolate Squares	152
162)	Chocolate and Raisin Cookie Bars	153
163)	Almond Granola Bars	153
164)	Coconut Cookies	**Error! Bookmark not defined.**
165)	Raw Walnut and Berry Cake	**Error! Bookmark not defined.**

AUTHOR BIOGRAPHY 154

CONCLUSIONS 156

© **Copyright 2021 - All rights reserved.**
The content contained within this book may not be reproduced, duplicated or transmitted without direct written permission from the author or the publisher.

Under no circumstances will any blame or legal responsibility be held against the publisher, or author, for any damages, reparation, or monetary loss due to the information contained within this book, either directly or indirectly.

Legal Notice:
This book is copyright protected. It is only for personal use. You cannot amend, distribute, sell, use, quote or paraphrase any part, or the content within this book, without the consent of the author or publisher.

Disclaimer Notice:
Please note the information contained within this document is for educational and entertainment purposes only. All effort has been executed to present accurate, up to date, reliable, complete information. No warranties of any kind are declared or implied. Readers acknowledge that the author is not engaged in the rendering of legal, financial, medical or professional advice. The content within this book has been de-rived from various sources. Please consult a licensed professional before attempting any techniques out-lined in this book.

By reading this document, the reader agrees that under no circumstances is the author responsible for any losses, direct or indirect, that are incurred as a result of the use of the information contained within this document, including, but not limited to, errors, omissions, or inaccuracies.

PART 2- INTRODUCTION to PLANT-BASED DIET

I've been on a primarily plant-based diet for a couple of years now, and I feel happy, energetic, and full of life. That's why I'm taking this opportunity to share my experiences with you through this cookbook.

This Plant-Based Cookbook comes from a deep place of passion and teaching where I guide those who diet regularly and beginners who want to transition to the plant-based lifestyle on its importance in today's age. It considers a trendy eating style, busy schedules, and tasty ideas to ensure that each recipe produced is not dull but delicious enough to enjoy cooking and eating.

My suggestion is to give the recipes a direct dive and enjoy all the delicious goodness that awaits you.

While the plant-based diet may seem torn between the vegetarian and vegan diets, it is neither. It is not a diet but a healthy lifestyle.

Unsurprisingly, an extensive discussion argues that the plant-based diet is either vegan (which is plant-centric) or vegetarian (which accommodates a certain amount of animal foods). Both cases are incorrect, however. The plant-based diet uses plant-based foods and strongly rejects processed foods such as white rice and added sugars. On the other hand, vegan and vegetarian diets allow some processed foods.

In this book, my goal is to present you with plant-based recipes in their healthiest form. The cookbook seeks to guide you. Beginners to the plant-based diet especially appreciate the essentials of whole plant foods, giving you flexible options and various cooking combinations.

Benefits of the plant-based diet

Plant-based foods are an excellent source of many nutrients that boost the body's metabolism in many ways. In addition, they are easy to digest due to their rich antioxidant content.

- Reduced risk of heart disease

Processed and animal foods are culprits of many heart diseases. The whole plant-based diet is better at nourishing the body with essential nutrients, improving the heart's function of producing and transporting blood to and from various parts of the body.

- Prevents and cures diabetes

Plant-based foods are excellent at reducing high blood sugar. Many studies that compared a vegetarian and vegan diet to a regular meat-filled diet showed that a diet with more plant-based foods reduced the risk of diabetes by 50%.

- An improved cognitive inclination

Fruits and vegetables are excellent for cleansing and increasing metabolism. They release a high number of plant compounds and antioxidants that slow or prevent cognitive decline. On a plant-based diet, the brain is boosted with sustainable energy, promoting sharp memory, language, thinking, and judgment skills.

- Rapid weight loss

A diet high in animal foods is known to promote weight gain. However, switching to a plant-based diet helps the body get rid of fat walls quickly, which results in rapid weight loss.

What to eat in a Plant-Based Lifestyle and PB Swaps

- Fruits - consume a wide range of fruits, whether fresh, dried, boiled, pureed, etc.

- Vegetables - all vegetables are permissible in the plant-based diet. They also provide plenty of essential vitamins and minerals for the body.

- Legumes are an excellent source of plant-based protein and fiber. Fiber is a nutrient that many people lack, and it is essential to increase its content in the body.

- Whole grains provide the body with nutrients such as selenium, copper, and magnesium. Meanwhile, they are rich in fiber when consumed in their whole-grain form. Avoid processed flours, rice, pasta, and bread in your plant-based diet, but consume brown rice, whole-wheat pasta, whole wheat bread, oats, barley, buckwheat, rye, quinoa spelled.

- Walnuts and nut butter - Walnuts are an essential source of selenium, vitamin E, and plant-based protein. They are excellent additions to desserts, smoothies, and snacks.

- Seeds are rich in calcium, vitamins, and healthy fats. Consume chia seeds, hemp seeds, flax seeds, pumpkin seeds, sunflower seeds, sesame seeds, etc.

- Healthy Oils and Fats - Plants offer a few options of healthy, fragrant oils and fats that are perfect for cooking, frying, sautéing, etc. They serve as an excellent substitute for dairy products and are rich in omega-3 fatty acids. Use olive oil, avocado, canola oil, walnuts, peanuts, hemp seeds, flax seeds, chia seeds, cashews, coconut oil.

- Plant-based milk, cream, and cheese - going plant-based doesn't mean staying away from creamy, milky, cheesy foods. You can instead plant-based alternatives using almond milk, soy milk, rice milk, cashew milk, coconut milk, coconut cream, cashew cream, hemp milk, oat milk.

- Plant-based meats - Have tofu, tempeh, seitan.

- Spices, herbs, and seasonings - All plant-based spices, herbs, and seasonings are permissible in the plant-based diet. Use basil example, turmeric, curry, black pepper, rosemary, oregano, thyme, sage, marjoram, salt, salsa, soy sauce, nutritional yeast, vinegar, homemade BBQ sauce, a homemade plant-based mayonnaise, etc.

- Beverages - You can drink coffee, sparkling water, tea, smoothies, etc.

FOOD TO AVOID

It has been established that all animal foods are not allowed in the plant-based diet, but other products are not allowed in a plant-based diet. Here is a detailed list:
- Animal meat: poultry, seafood, pork, lamb, and beef
- Butter, ghee, and other solid animal fats
- All processed foods
- Sugary foods such as cookies, cakes, and pastries
- All refined white carbohydrates
- Processed vegan and vegetarian alternatives that may contain added salt or sugar
- Excessive salt
- Fried foods

EIGHT FOOD-BASED MISTAKES
Without a clear understanding of the diet, people can make some mistakes while following a plant-based diet. This is mainly due to the subtle differences between the ingredients. The following are common food mistakes that people usually make and the different ways to avoid them:

BREAD
There are countless varieties of bread available today. While all loaves are made primarily from a basic flour batter, many additional ingredients can compromise the plant-based diet. The addition of butter, animal milk, fat or other animal products, or an excess of sugar and salt can make bread unsuitable for a plant-based diet. Be sure to double-check the ingredients in store-bought bread or make your bread at home using only vegan ingredients.

BROTH FOR SOUPS
Broths are commonly used in soups and curries, but most are liquid extracts of bones, meat, and vegetables. Because chicken and beef broths are usually used in popular soup recipes, people also use them in a plant-based diet. Vegetable broths and stocks should be used instead. The broth gets most of its nutrients and fat from the meat or bones in which it is cooked, so only vegetable broths are recommended for this diet.

PASTA
Whole wheat or basic flour pasta is an excellent option for enjoying some flavor and variety in your plant-based diet. Adding pasta to your plant-based menu is not harmful, but if the same pasta is cooked with animal ingredients, it is not suitable for this diet. Plant-based pasta recipes, including zucchini spaghetti, are also an excellent option for this diet.

ORANGE JUICE
Freshly squeezed organic orange juice is not nasty for the plant-based diet. It is a good source of vitamin C. However, when the juice is processed to add additional nutrients, the problem begins. Some companies add vitamin D2 or D3 to the juice. While vitamin D2 comes from plants, vitamin D3 is an animal-based vitamin not allowed in a plant-based diet. Read labels and do your research to avoid such products. It's best to rely on homemade, freshly squeezed juices rather than store-bought ones.

GRANOLA
Granola comes in a wide variety. Because of the diversity of ingredients used in different granola recipes, a person on a plant-based diet should be more careful in their selection. Granola may contain dairy products such as milk, butter, or eggs. These should be avoided completely. Instead, choose one made from oats, nuts, seeds, and vegetable fats while following this diet.

CREAMS AND CUSTARDS
Since all creams and cream cheeses are made from animal milk, they are prohibited in a plant-based diet, even in small amounts. Instead, non-dairy, plant-based creams should be used. Ointments made from soy or coconut milk taste good and have a rich, thick texture, just like other creams.

CHEESE
Cheese is a staple in most diets, but they are animal-based and now allowed, as mentioned above. This is where vegan cheeses come in. These cheeses are made with plant-based ingredients, including soy, nuts, tapioca, coconut, root vegetables, or aquafaba. Like dairy cheese, vegan cheese varies in shape, texture, and taste but provides a good substitute for animal-based cheese.

VEGAN SAUSAGES AND BURGERS
Burgers and sausages are commonly enjoyed and hard to pass up. Fortunately, now both burgers and sausages are available in plant-based varieties. These burgers and sausages look more like meat-based burgers and sausages but are made of shredded vegetables and batter. Always opt for these varieties while following a plant-based diet.

BREAKFAST

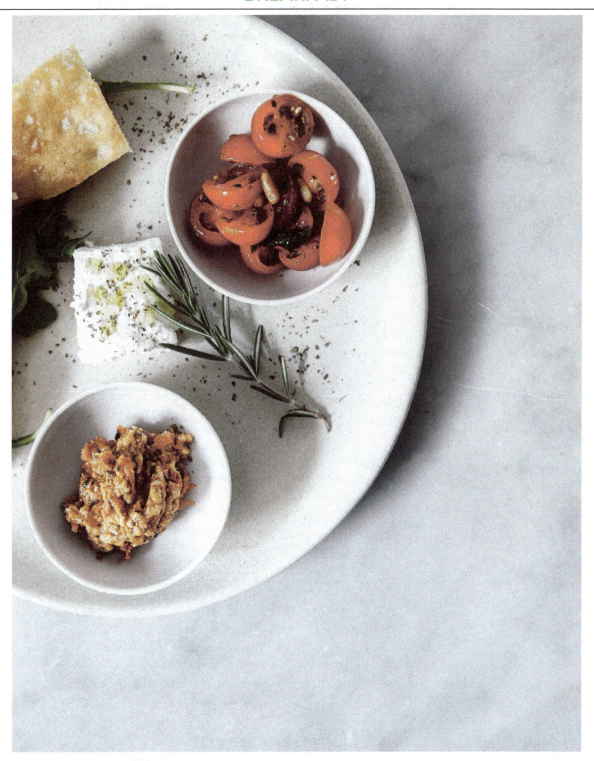

126) BANANA PANCAKES

Preparation Time: 25 minutes
Preparation Time:
Preparation Time: 4

Ingredients:

- ✓ 2 tbsp ground flaxseeds
- ✓ 1/2 cup oat flour
- ✓ 1/2 cup coconut flour
- ✓ 1/2 cup instant oats
- ✓ 1 tsp baking powder
- ✓ 1/4 tsp kosher salt

Ingredients:

- ✓ 1/4 tsp ground cardamom
- ✓ 1/4 tsp ground cinnamon
- ✓ 1/2 tsp coconut extract
- ✓ 1 cup banana
- ✓ 2 tbsp coconut oil, at room temperature

Ingredients:

- ❖ To make the "flax" egg, in a small mixing dish, whisk 2 tbsp of the ground flaxseeds with 4 tbsp of the water. Let it sit for at least 15 minutes.
- ❖ In a mixing bowl, thoroughly combine the flour, oats, baking powder and spices. Add in the flax egg and mashed banana. Mix until everything is well incorporated.
- ❖ Heat 1/2 tbsp of the coconut oil in a frying pan over medium-low flame. Spoon about 1/4 cup of the batter into the frying pan; fry your pancake for approximately 3 minutes per side.
- ❖ Repeat until you run out of batter. Serve with your favorite fixings and enjoy

127) PESTO BREAD

Preparation Time: 35 minutes
Preparation Time:
Preparation Time: 6

Ingredients:

- ✓ 1 ½ cups grated plant-based mozzarella cheese
- ✓ 1 tbsp flax seed powder
- ✓ 4 tbsp coconut flour
- ✓ ½ cup almond flour
- ✓ ½ tsp salt

Ingredients:

- ✓ 1 tsp baking powder
- ✓ 5 tbsp plant butter
- ✓ 2 oz pesto
- ✓ Olive oil for brushing

Ingredients:

- ❖ First, mix the flax seed powder with 3 tbsp water in a bowl, and set aside to soak for 5 minutes.
- ❖ Preheat oven to 350 F and line a baking sheet with parchment paper. In a bowl, evenly combine the coconut flour, almond flour, salt, and baking powder. Melt the plant butter and cheese in a deep skillet over medium heat and stir in the vegan "flax egg." Mix in the flour mixture until a firm dough forms.
- ❖ Turn the heat off, transfer the mixture in between two parchment papers, and then use a rolling pin to flatten out the dough of about an inch's thickness.
- ❖ Remove the parchment paper on top and spread the pesto all over the dough. Now, use a knife to cut the dough into strips, twist each piece, and place it on the baking sheet.
- ❖ Brush with olive oil and bake for 15 to 20 minutes until golden brown.
- ❖ Remove the bread twist; allow cooling for a few minutes, and serve with warm almond milk

128) CLASSIC FRENCH TOASTS

Preparation Time: 16 minutes
Preparation Time:
Preparation Time: 2

The Plant-Based for Athlete

Ingredients:

- 4 tbsp flaxseed
- 1 tsp plant butter
- 2 tbsp coconut flour
- 2 tbsp almond flour
- 1 ½ tsp baking powder
- A pinch of salt

Ingredients:

- 2 tbsp coconut cream
- 2 tbsp coconut milk whipping cream
- ½ tsp cinnamon powder
- 2 tbsp plant butter

Ingredients:

- For the vegan "flax egg," whisk flax seed powder and 12 tbsp water in two separate bowls and leave to soak for 5 minutes.
- Grease a glass dish (for the microwave) with 1 tsp plant butter. In another bowl, mix coconut flour, almond flour, baking powder, and salt.
- When the flaxseed egg is ready, whisk one portion with the coconut cream and add the mixture to the dry ingredients. Continue whisking until the mixture is smooth with no lumps. Pour the dough into the glass dish and microwave for 2 minutes or until the bread's middle part is done. Take out and allow the bread to cool. Remove the bread and slice in half. Return to the glass dish.
- Whisk the remaining vegan "flax egg" with the coconut milk whipping cream until well combined. Pour the mixture over the bread slices and leave to soak. Turn the bread a few times to soak in as much of the batter. Melt 2 tbsp of the plant butter in a frying pan and fry the bread slices on both sides. Transfer to a serving plate, sprinkle with cinnamon powder and serve

129) **CREAMY BREAD WITH SESAME**

Preparation Time: 40 minutes   **Preparation Time:**   **Preparation Time:** 6

Ingredients:

- 4 tbsp flax seed powder
- 2/3 cup cashew cream cheese
- 4 tbsp sesame oil + for brushing
- 1 cup coconut flour

Ingredients:

- 2 tbsp psyllium husk powder
- 1 tsp salt
- 1 tsp baking powder
- 1 tbsp sesame seeds

Ingredients:

- In a bowl, mix the flax seed powder with 1 ½ cups water until smoothly combined and set aside to soak for 5 minutes. Preheat oven to 400 F. When the vegan "flax egg" is ready, beat in the cream cheese and sesame oil until well mixed.
- Whisk in the coconut flour, psyllium husk powder, salt, and baking powder until adequately blended.
- Grease a 9 x 5 inches baking tray with cooking spray, and spread the dough in the tray. Allow the mixture to stand for 5 minutes and then brush with some sesame oil.
- Sprinkle with the sesame seeds and bake the dough for 30 minutes or until golden brown on top and set within. Take out the bread and allow cooling for a few minutes. Slice and serve

130) **DIFFERENT SEEDS BREAD**

Preparation Time: 55 minutes   **Preparation Time:**   **Preparation Time:** 6

The Plant-Based for Athlete

Ingredients:

- ✓ 3 tbsp ground flax seeds
- ✓ ¾ cup coconut flour
- ✓ 1 cup almond flour
- ✓ 3 tsp baking powder
- ✓ 5 tbsp sesame seeds
- ✓ ½ cup chia seeds
- ✓ 1 tsp ground caraway seeds
- ✓ 1 tsp hemp seeds

Ingredients:

- ✓ ¼ cup psyllium husk powder
- ✓ 1 tsp salt
- ✓ 2/3 cup cashew cream cheese
- ✓ ½ cup melted coconut oil
- ✓ ¾ cup coconut cream
- ✓ 1 tbsp poppy seeds

Ingredients:

- ❖ Preheat oven to 350 F and line a loaf pan with parchment paper.
- ❖ For the vegan "flax egg," whisk flax seed powder with ½ cup of water and let the mixture sit to soak for 5 minutes. In a bowl, evenly combine the coconut flour, almond flour, baking powder, sesame seeds, chia seeds, ground caraway seeds, hemp seeds, psyllium husk powder, and salt.
- ❖ In another bowl, use an electric hand mixer to whisk the cream cheese, coconut oil, coconut whipping cream, and vegan "flax egg." Pour the liquid ingredients into the dry ingredients, and continue whisking with the hand mixer until a dough forms. Transfer the dough to the loaf pan, sprinkle with poppy seeds, and bake in the oven for 45 minutes or until a knife inserted into the bread comes out clean. Remove the parchment paper with the bread, and allow cooling on a rack

131) NAAN BREAD

Preparation Time: 25 minutes

Preparation Time:

Preparation Time: 6

Ingredients:

- ✓ ¾ cup almond flour
- ✓ 2 tbsp psyllium husk powder
- ✓ ½ tsp salt
- ✓ ½ tsp baking powder
- ✓ 1/3 cup olive oil

Ingredients:

- ✓ Plant butter for frying
- ✓ 4 oz plant butter
- ✓ 2 garlic cloves, minced

Ingredients:

- ❖ In a bowl, mix the almond flour, psyllium husk powder, salt, and baking powder.
- ❖ Mix in some olive oil and 2 cups of boiling water to combine the ingredients, like a thick porridge. Stir thoroughly and allow the dough to rise for 5 minutes.
- ❖ Divide the dough into 6 to 8 pieces and mold into balls. Place the balls on parchment paper and flatten with your hands.
- ❖ Melt the plant butter in a frying pan and fry the naan on both sides to have a beautiful, golden color. Transfer the naan to a plate and keep warm in the oven. For the garlic butter, add the remaining plant butter to the frying pan and sauté the garlic until fragrant, about 3 minutes. Pour the garlic butter into a bowl and serve as a dip along with the naan

132) MUSHROOM AND SPINACH CHICKPEA OMELETTE

Preparation Time: 25 minutes

Servings: 4

Ingredients:

- 1 cup chickpea flour
- ½ tsp onion powder
- ½ tsp garlic powder
- ¼ tsp white pepper
- 1/3 cup nutritional yeast
- ½ tsp baking soda
- 1 green bell pepper, chopped
- 3 scallions, chopped
- 1 cup sautéed button mushrooms
- ½ cup chopped fresh spinach
- 1 cup halved cherry tomatoes
- 1 tbsp fresh parsley leaves

Directions:

- In a medium bowl, mix the chickpea flour, onion powder, garlic powder, white pepper, nutritional yeast, and baking soda until well combined. Heat a medium skillet over medium heat and add a quarter of the batter. Swirl the pan to spread the batter across the pan. Scatter a quarter each of the bell pepper, scallions, mushrooms, and spinach on top and cook until the bottom part of the omelet sets, 1-2 minutes.
- Carefully flip the omelet and cook the other side until set and golden brown. Transfer the omelet to a plate and make the remaining omelets. Serve the omelet with the tomatoes and garnish with the parsley leaves

133) COCONUT-RASPBERRY PANCAKES

Preparation Time: 25 minutes
Servings: 4

Ingredients:

- 2 tbsp flax seed powder
- ½ cup coconut milk
- ¼ cup fresh raspberries, mashed
- ½ cup oat flour
- 1 tsp baking soda
- A pinch salt
- 1 tbsp coconut sugar
- 2 tbsp pure date syrup
- ½ tsp cinnamon powder
- 2 tbsp unsweetened coconut flakes
- 2 tsp plant butter
- Fresh raspberries for garnishing

Directions:

- In a medium bowl, mix the flax seed powder with the 6 tbsp water and thicken for 5 minutes. Mix in coconut milk and raspberries. Add the oat flour, baking soda, salt, coconut sugar, date syrup, and cinnamon powder. Fold in the coconut flakes until well combined.
- Working in batches, melt a quarter of the butter in a non-stick skillet and add ¼ cup of the batter. Cook until set beneath and golden brown, 2 minutes. Flip the pancake and cook on the other side until set and golden brown, 2 minutes. Transfer to a plate and make the remaining pancakes using the rest of the ingredients in the same proportions. Garnish the pancakes with some raspberries and serve warm

134) BLUEBERRY-CHIA PUDDING

Preparation Time: 5 minutes + chilling time
Servings: 2

Ingredients:

- ¾ cup coconut milk
- ½ tsp vanilla extract
- ½ cup blueberries
- 2 tbsp chia seeds
- Chopped walnuts to garnish

Directions:

- In a blender, pour the coconut milk, vanilla extract, and half of the blueberries. Process the ingredients at high speed until the blueberries have incorporated into the liquid.
- Open the blender and mix in the chia seeds. Share the mixture into two breakfast jars, cover, and

refrigerate for 4 hours to allow the mixture to gel. Garnish the pudding with the remaining blueberries and walnuts. Serve immediately

135) POTATO AND CAULIFLOWER BROWNS

Preparation Time: 35 minutes
Servings: 4

Ingredients:

- 3 tbsp flax seed powder
- 2 large potatoes, shredded
- 1 big head cauliflower, riced
- ½ white onion, grated
- Salt and black pepper to taste
- 4 tbsp plant butter

Directions:

- In a medium bowl, mix the flaxseed powder and 9 tbsp water. Allow thickening for 5 minutes for the vegan "flax egg." Add the potatoes, cauliflower, onion, salt, and black pepper to the vegan "flax egg" and mix until well combined. Allow sitting for 5 minutes to thicken.
- Working in batches, melt 1 tbsp of plant butter in a non-stick skillet and add 4 scoops of the hashbrown mixture to the skillet. Make sure to have 1 to 2-inch intervals between each scoop.
- Use the spoon to flatten the batter and cook until compacted and golden brown on the bottom part, 2 minutes. Flip the hashbrowns and cook further for 2 minutes or until the vegetable cook and is golden brown. Transfer to a paper-towel-lined plate to drain grease. Make the remaining hashbrowns using the remaining ingredients. Serve warm

136) PISTACHIOS-PUMPKIN CAKE

Preparation Time: 70 minutes **Servings:** 4

Ingredients:

- 2 tbsp flaxseed powder
- 3 tbsp vegetable oil
- ¾ cup canned pumpkin puree
- ½ cup pure corn syrup
- 3 tbsp pure date sugar
- 1 ½ cups whole-wheat flour
- ½ tsp cinnamon powder
- ½ tsp baking powder
- ¼ tsp cloves powder
- ½ tsp allspice powder
- ½ tsp nutmeg powder
- 2 tbsp chopped pistachios

Directions:

- Preheat the oven to 350 F and lightly coat an 8 x 4-inch loaf pan with cooking spray. In a bowl, mix the flax seed powder with 6 tbsp water and allow thickening for 5 minutes to make the vegan "flax egg."
- In a bowl, whisk the vegetable oil, pumpkin puree, corn syrup, date sugar, and vegan "flax egg." In another bowl, mix the flour, cinnamon powder, baking powder, cloves powder, allspice powder, and nutmeg powder. Add this mixture to the wet batter and mix until well combined. Pour the batter into the loaf pan, sprinkle the pistachios on top, and gently press the nuts onto the batter to stick.
- Bake in the oven for 50-55 minutes or until a toothpick inserted into the cake comes out clean. Remove the cake onto a wire rack, allow cooling, slice, and serve

137) BELL PEPPER WITH SCRAMBLED TOFU

Preparation Time: 20 minutes **Servings:** 4

Ingredients:

- 2 tbsp plant butter, for frying
- 1 (14 oz) pack firm tofu, crumbled
- 1 red bell pepper, chopped
- 1 green bell pepper, chopped
- 1 tomato, finely chopped
- 2 tbsp chopped fresh green onions
- Salt and black pepper to taste
- 1 tsp turmeric powder
- 1 tsp Creole seasoning
- ½ cup chopped baby kale
- ¼ cup grated plant-based Parmesan

Directions:

- Melt the plant butter in a skillet over medium heat and add the tofu. Cook with occasional stirring until the tofu is light golden brown while, making sure not to break the tofu into tiny bits but to have scrambled egg resemblance, 5 minutes.
- Stir in the bell peppers, tomato, green onions, salt, black pepper, turmeric powder, and Creole seasoning. Sauté until the vegetables soften, 5 minutes. Mix in the kale to wilt, 3 minutes and then half of the plant-based Parmesan cheese.
- Allow melting for 1 to 2 minutes and then turn the heat off. Top with the remaining cheese and serve warm

138) ORIGINAL FRENCH TOAST

Preparation Time: 20 minutes **Servings:** 2

Ingredients:

- 1 tbsp ground flax seeds
- 1 cup coconut milk
- 1/2 tsp vanilla paste
- A pinch of sea salt
- A pinch of grated nutmeg
- 1/2 tsp ground cinnamon
- 1/4 tsp ground cloves
- 1 tbsp agave syrup
- 4 slices bread

Directions:

- In a mixing bowl, thoroughly combine the flax seeds, coconut milk, vanilla, salt, nutmeg, cinnamon, cloves and agave syrup.
- Dredge each slice of bread into the milk mixture until well coated on all sides.
- Preheat an electric griddle to medium heat and lightly oil it with a nonstick cooking spray.
- Cook each slice of bread on the preheated griddle for about 3 minutes per side until golden brown.
- Enjoy

139) FRYBREAD WITH PEANUT BUTTER AND JAM

Preparation Time: 20 minutes **Servings:** 3

Ingredients:

- 1 cup all-purpose flour
- 1/2 tsp baking powder
- 1/2 tsp sea salt
- 1 tsp coconut sugar
- 1/2 cup warm water
- 3 tsp olive oil
- 3 tbsp peanut butter
- 3 tbsp raspberry jam

Directions:

- Thoroughly combine the flour, baking powder, salt and sugar. Gradually add in the water until the dough comes together.
- Divide the dough into three balls; flatten each ball to create circles.
- Heat 1 tsp of the olive oil in a frying pan over a moderate flame. Fry the first bread for about 9 minutes or until golden brown. Repeat with the remaining oil and dough.
- Serve the frybread with the peanut butter and raspberry jam. Enjoy

The Plant-Based for Athlete

140) PUDDING WITH SULTANAS ON CIABATTA BREAD

Preparation Time: 2 hours 10 minutes

Servings: 4

Ingredients:

- 2 cups coconut milk, unsweetened
- 1/2 cup agave syrup
- 1 tbsp coconut oil
- 1/2 tsp vanilla essence
- 1/2 tsp ground cardamom
- 1/4 tsp ground cloves
- 1/2 tsp ground cinnamon
- 1/4 tsp Himalayan salt
- 3/4 pound stale ciabatta bread, cubed
- 1/2 cup sultana raisins

Directions:

- In a mixing bowl, combine the coconut milk, agave syrup, coconut oil, vanilla, cardamom, ground cloves, cinnamon and Himalayan salt.
- Add the bread cubes to the custard mixture and stir to combine well. Fold in the sultana raisins and allow it to rest for about 1 hour on a counter.
- Then, spoon the mixture into a lightly oiled casserole dish.
- Bake in the preheated oven at 350 degrees F for about 1 hour or until the top is golden brown.
- Place the bread pudding on a wire rack for 10 minutes before slicing and serving

141) VEGAN BANH MI

Preparation Time: 35 minutes

Servings: 4

Ingredients:

- 1/2 cup rice vinegar
- 1/4 cup water
- 1/4 cup white sugar
- 2 carrots, cut into 1/16-inch-thick matchsticks
- 1/2 cup white (daikon) radish, cut into 1/16-inch-thick matchsticks
- 1 white onion, thinly sliced
- 2 tbsp olive oil
- 12 ounces firm tofu, cut into sticks
- 1/4 cup vegan mayonnaise
- 1 ½ tbsp soy sauce
- 2 cloves garlic, minced
- 1/4 cup fresh parsley, chopped
- Kosher salt and ground black pepper, to taste
- 2 standard French baguettes, cut into four pieces
- 4 tbsp fresh cilantro, chopped
- 4 lime wedges

Directions:

- Bring the rice vinegar, water and sugar to a boil and stir until the sugar has dissolved, about 1 minute. Allow it to cool.
- Pour the cooled vinegar mixture over the carrot, daikon radish and onion; allow the vegetables to marinate for at least 30 minutes.
- While the vegetables are marinating, heat the olive oil in a frying pan over medium-high heat. Once hot, add the tofu and sauté for 8 minutes, stirring occasionally to promote even cooking.
- Then, mix the mayo, soy sauce, garlic, parsley, salt and ground black pepper in a small bowl.
- Slice each piece of the baguette in half the long way Then, toast the baguette halves under the preheated broiler for about 3 minutes.
- To assemble the banh mi sandwiches, spread each half of the toasted baguette with the mayonnaise mixture; fill the cavity of the bottom half of the bread with the fried tofu sticks, marinated vegetables and cilantro leaves.
- Lastly, squeeze the lime wedges over the filling and top with the other half of the baguette. Enjoy

142) BREAKFAST NUTTY OATMEAL MUFFINS

Preparation Time: 30 minutes

Servings: 9

Ingredients:

- 1 ½ cups rolled oats
- 1/2 cup shredded coconut, unsweetened
- 3/4 tsp baking powder
- 1/4 tsp salt
- 1/4 tsp vanilla extract
- 1/4 tsp coconut extract
- 1/4 tsp grated nutmeg
- 1/2 tsp cardamom
- 3/4 cup coconut milk
- 1/3 cup canned pumpkin
- 1/4 cup agave syrup
- 1/4 cup golden raisins
- 1/4 cup pecans, chopped

Directions:

- Begin by preheating your oven to 360 degrees F. Spritz a muffin tin with a nonstick cooking oil.
- In a mixing bowl, thoroughly combine all the ingredients, except for the raisins and pecans.
- Fold in the raisins and pecans and scrape the batter into the prepared muffin tin.
- Bake your muffins for about 25 minutes or until the top is set. Enjoy

143) SMOOTHIE BOWL OF RASPBERRY AND CHIA

Preparation Time: 10 minutes **Servings:** 2

Ingredients:

- 1 cup coconut milk
- 2 small-sized bananas, peeled
- 1 ½ cups raspberries, fresh or frozen
- 2 dates, pitted
- 1 tbsp coconut flakes
- 1 tbsp pepitas
- 2 tbsp chia seeds

Directions:

- In your blender or food processor, mix the coconut milk with the bananas, raspberries and dates.
- Process until creamy and smooth. Divide the smoothie between two bowls.
- Top each smoothie bowl with the coconut flakes, pepitas and chia seeds. Enjoy

144) BREAKFAST OATS WITH WALNUTS AND CURRANTS

Preparation Time: 10 minutes **Servings:** 2

Ingredients:

- 1 cup water
- 1 ½ cups oat milk
- 1 ½ cups rolled oats
- A pinch of salt
- A pinch of grated nutmeg
- 1/4 tsp cardamom
- 1 handful walnuts, roughly chopped
- 4 tbsp dried currants

Directions:

- In a deep saucepan, bring the water and milk to a rolling boil. Add in the oats, cover the saucepan and turn the heat to medium.
- Add in the salt, nutmeg and cardamom. Continue to cook for about 12 to 13 minutes more, stirring occasionally.
- Spoon the mixture into serving bowls; top with walnuts and currants. Enjoy

145) APPLESAUCE PANCAKES WITH COCONUT

Preparation Time: 50 minutes **Servings:** 8

Ingredients:

- 1 ¼ cups whole-wheat flour
- 1 tsp baking powder
- 1/4 tsp sea salt
- 1/2 tsp ground cinnamon
- 3/4 cup oat milk
- 1/2 cup applesauce, unsweetened
- 2 tbsp coconut oil

Directions:

- In a mixing bowl, thoroughly combine the flour, baking powder, salt, sugar and spices. Gradually add in the milk and applesauce.
- Heat a frying pan over a moderately high flame and add a small amount of the coconut oil.

- ✓ 1/2 tsp coconut sugar
- ✓ 1/4 tsp ground cloves
- ✓ 1/4 tsp ground cardamom
- ✓ 8 tbsp coconut, shredded
- ✓ 8 tbsp pure maple syrup

- ❖ Once hot, pour the batter into the frying pan. Cook for approximately 3 minutes until the bubbles form; flip it and cook on the other side for 3 minutes longer until browned on the underside. Repeat with the remaining oil and batter.
- ❖ Serve with shredded coconut and maple syrup. Enjoy

146) VEGGIE PANINI

Preparation Time: 30 minutes

Servings: 4

Ingredients:

- ✓ 1 tbsp olive oil
- ✓ 1 cup sliced button mushrooms
- ✓ Salt and black pepper to taste
- ✓ 1 ripe avocado, sliced
- ✓ 2 tbsp freshly squeezed lemon juice
- ✓ 1 tbsp chopped parsley
- ✓ ½ tsp pure maple syrup
- ✓ 8 slices whole-wheat ciabatta
- ✓ 4 oz sliced plant-based Parmesan

Directions:

- ❖ Heat the olive oil in a medium skillet over medium heat and sauté the mushrooms until softened, 5 minutes. Season with salt and black pepper. Turn the heat off.
- ❖ Preheat a panini press to medium heat, 3 to 5 minutes. Mash the avocado in a medium bowl and mix in the lemon juice, parsley, and maple syrup. Spread the mixture on 4 bread slices, divide the mushrooms and plant-based Parmesan cheese on top.
- ❖ Cover with the other bread slices and brush the top with olive oil. Grill the sandwiches one after another in the heated press until golden brown, and the cheese is melted.
- ❖ Serve

147) CHEDDAR GRITS AND SOY CHORIZO

Preparation Time: 25 minutes **Servings:** 6

Ingredients:

- ✓ 1 cup quick-cooking grits
- ✓ ½ cup grated plant-based cheddar
- ✓ 2 tbsp peanut butter
- ✓ 1 cup soy chorizo, chopped
- ✓ 1 cup corn kernels
- ✓ 2 cups vegetable broth

Directions:

- ❖ Preheat oven to 380 F.
- ❖ Pour the broth in a pot and bring to a boil over medium heat. Stir in salt and grits. Lower the heat and cook until the grits are thickened, stirring often. Turn the heat off, put in the plant-based cheddar cheese, peanut butter, soy chorizo, and corn and mix well.
- ❖ Spread the mixture into a greased baking dish and bake for 45 minutes until slightly puffed and golden brown. Serve right away

148) VANILLA CREPES AND BERRY CREAM COMPOTE TOPPING

Preparation Time: 35 minutes **Servings:** 4

Ingredients:

- ✓ For the berry cream:
- ✓ 2 tbsp plant butter
- ✓ 2 tbsp pure date sugar
- ✓ 1 tsp vanilla extract
- ✓ ½ cup fresh blueberries
- ✓ ½ cup fresh raspberries
- ✓ ½ cup whipped coconut cream
- ✓ For the crepes:
- ✓ 2 tbsp flax seed powder
- ✓ 1 tsp vanilla extract
- ✓ 1 tsp pure date sugar
- ✓ ¼ tsp salt
- ✓ 2 cups almond flour
- ✓ 1 ½ cups almond milk
- ✓ 1 ½ cups water
- ✓ 3 tbsp plant butter for frying

Directions:

- ❖ Melt butter in a pot over low heat and mix in the date sugar, and vanilla. Cook until the sugar melts and then toss in berries. Allow softening for 2-3 minutes. Set aside to cool.
- ❖ In a medium bowl, mix the flax seed powder with 6 tbsp water and allow to thicken for 5 minutes to make the vegan "flax egg." Whisk in vanilla, date sugar, and salt. Pour in a quarter cup of almond flour and whisk, then a quarter cup of almond milk, and mix until no lumps remain. Repeat the mixing process with the remaining almond flour and almond milk in the same quantities until exhausted.
- ❖ Mix in 1 cup of water until the mixture is runny like that of pancakes and add the remaining water until it is lighter. Brush a large non-stick skillet with some butter and place over medium heat to melt. Pour 1 tbsp of the batter into the pan and swirl the skillet quickly and all around to coat the pan with the batter. Cook until the batter is dry and golden brown beneath, about 30 seconds.
- ❖ Use a spatula to carefully flip the crepe and cook the other side until golden brown too. Fold the crepe onto a plate and set aside. Repeat making more crepes with the remaining batter until exhausted. Plate the crepes, top with the whipped coconut cream and the berry compote. Serve immediately

149) STRAWBERRY AND PECAN BREAKFAST

Preparation Time: 15 minutes **Servings:** 2

Ingredients:

- 1 (14-oz) can coconut milk, refrigerated overnight
- 1 cup granola
- ½ cup pecans, chopped
- 1 cup sliced strawberries

Directions:

- Drain the coconut milk liquid. Layer the coconut milk solids, granola, and strawberries in small glasses. Top with chopped pecans and serve right away

150) GRANOLA WITH HAZELNUTS AND ORANGE

Preparation Time: 50 minutes **Servings:** 5

Ingredients:

- 2 cups rolled oats
- ¾ cup whole-wheat flour
- 1 tbsp ground cinnamon
- 1 tsp ground ginger
- ½ cup sunflower seeds
- ½ cup hazelnuts, chopped
- ½ cup pumpkin seeds
- ½ cup shredded coconut
- 1 ¼ cups orange juice
- ½ cup dried cherries
- ½ cup goji berries

Directions:

- Preheat oven to 350 F.
- In a bowl, combine the oats, flour, cinnamon, ginger, sunflower seeds, hazelnuts, pumpkin seeds, and coconut. Pour in the orange juice, toss to mix well.
- Transfer to a baking sheet and bake for 15 minutes. Turn the granola and continue baking until it is crunchy, about 30 minutes. Stir in the cherries and goji berries and store in the fridge for up to 14 days

151) ORANGE CREPES

Preparation Time: 30 minutes **Servings:** 4

Ingredients:

- 2 tbsp flax seed powder
- 1 tsp vanilla extract
- 1 tsp pure date sugar
- ¼ tsp salt
- 2 cups almond flour
- 1 ½ cups oat milk
- ½ cup melted plant butter
- 3 tbsp fresh orange juice
- 3 tbsp plant butter for frying

Directions:

- In a medium bowl, mix the flax seed powder with 6 tbsp water and allow thickening for 5 minutes to make the vegan "flax egg." Whisk in the vanilla, date sugar, and salt.
- Pour in a quarter cup of almond flour and whisk, then a quarter cup of oat milk, and mix until no lumps remain. Repeat the mixing process with the remaining almond flour and almond milk in the same quantities until exhausted.
- Mix in the plant butter, orange juice, and half of the water until the mixture is runny like pancakes. Add the remaining water until the mixture is lighter. Brush a non-stick skillet with some butter and place over medium heat to melt.
- Pour 1 tbsp of the batter into the pan and swirl the skillet quickly and all around to coat the pan with the batter. Cook until the batter is dry and golden brown beneath, about 30 seconds.
- Use a spatula to flip the crepe and cook the other side until golden brown too. Fold the crepe onto a plate and set aside. Repeat making more crepes with the remaining batter until exhausted. Drizzle some maple syrup on the crepes and serve

152) OAT BREAD WITH COCONUT

Preparation Time: 50 minutes **Servings:** 4

Ingredients:

- 4 cups whole-wheat flour
- ¼ tsp salt
- ½ cup rolled oats
- 1 tsp baking soda
- 1 ¾ cups coconut milk, thick
- 2 tbsp pure maple syrup

Directions:

- Preheat the oven to 400 F.
- In a bowl, mix flour, salt, oats, and baking soda. Add in coconut milk and maple syrup and whisk until dough forms. Dust your hands with some flour and knead the dough into a ball. Shape the dough into a circle and place on a baking sheet.
- Cut a deep cross on the dough and bake in the oven for 15 minutes at 450 F. Reduce the temperature to 400 F and bake further for 20 to 25 minutes or until a hollow sound is made when the bottom of the bread is tapped. Slice and serve

153) BOWL WITH BLACK BEANS AND SPICY QUINOA

Preparation Time: 25 minutes **Servings:** 4

Ingredients:

- 1 cup brown quinoa, rinsed
- 3 tbsp plant-based yogurt
- ½ lime, juiced
- 2 tbsp chopped fresh cilantro
- 1 (5 oz) can black beans, drained
- 3 tbsp tomato salsa
- ¼ avocado, sliced
- 2 radishes, shredded
- 1 tbsp pepitas (pumpkin seeds)

Directions:

- Cook the quinoa with 2 cups of slightly salted water in a medium pot over medium heat or until the liquid absorbs, 15 minutes. Spoon the quinoa into serving bowls and fluff with a fork.
- In a small bowl, mix the yogurt, lime juice, cilantro, and salt. Divide this mixture on the quinoa and top with the beans, salsa, avocado, radishes, and pepitas. Serve immediately

154) ALMOND AND RAISIN GRANOLA

Preparation Time: 20 minutes **Servings:** 8

Ingredients:

- 5 ½ cups old-fashioned oats
- 1 ½ cups chopped walnuts
- ½ cup shelled sunflower seeds
- 1 cup golden raisins
- 1 cup shaved almonds
- 1 cup pure maple syrup
- ½ tsp ground cinnamon
- ¼ tsp ground allspice
- A pinch of salt

Directions:

- Preheat oven to 325 F. In a baking dish, place the oats, walnuts, and sunflower seeds. Bake for 10 minutes.
- Lower the heat from the oven to 300 F. Stir in the raisins, almonds, maple syrup, cinnamon, allspice, and salt. Bake for an additional 15 minutes. Allow cooling before serving

155) PECAN AND PUMPKIN SEED OAT JARS

Preparation Time: 10 minutes + chilling time **Servings:** 5

Ingredients:

- 2 ½ cups old-fashioned rolled oats
- 5 tbsp pumpkin seeds
- 5 tbsp chopped pecans
- 5 cups unsweetened soy milk
- 2 ½ tsp agave syrup
- Salt to taste
- 1 tsp ground cardamom
- 1 tsp ground ginger

Directions:

- • In a bowl, put oats, pumpkin seeds, pecans, soy milk, agave syrup, salt, cardamom, and ginger and toss to combine. Divide the mixture between mason jars. Seal the lids and transfer to the fridge to soak for 10-12 hours

156) EASY APPLE MUFFINS

Preparation Time: 40 minutes **Servings:** 4

Ingredients:

- For the muffins:
- 1 flax seed powder + 3 tbsp water
- 1 ½ cups whole-wheat
- For topping:
- 1/3 cup whole-wheat flour
- ½ cup pure date sugar

Directions:

- Preheat oven to 400 F and grease 6 muffin cups with cooking spray. In a bowl, mix the flax seed powder with water and allow thickening for 5 minutes to make the vegan "flax egg."

The Plant-Based for Athlete

- flour
- ¾ cup pure date sugar
- 2 tsp baking powder
- ¼ tsp salt
- 1 tsp cinnamon powder
- 1/3 cup melted plant butter
- 1/3 cup flax milk
- 2 apples, chopped
- ½ cup cold plant butter, cubed
- 1 ½ tsp cinnamon powder

❖ In a bowl, mix flour, date sugar, baking powder, salt, and cinnamon powder. Whisk in the butter, vegan "flax egg," flax milk, and fold in the apples. Fill the muffin cups two-thirds way up with the batter.

❖ In a bowl, mix remaining flour, date sugar, cold butter, and cinnamon powder. Sprinkle the mixture on the muffin batter. Bake for 20 minutes. Remove the muffins onto a wire rack, allow cooling, and serve

157) ALMOND YOGURT WITH BERRIES AND WALNUTS

Preparation Time: 10 minutes   **Servings:** 4

Ingredients:

- 4 cups almond milk
- Dairy-Free yogurt, cold
- 2 tbsp pure malt syrup
- 2 cups mixed berries, chopped
- ¼ cup chopped toasted walnuts

Directions:

❖ In a medium bowl, mix the yogurt and malt syrup until well-combined. Divide the mixture into 4 breakfast bowls. Top with the berries and walnuts. Enjoy immediately

158) BREAKFAST BLUEBERRY MUESLI

Preparation Time: 10 minutes   **Servings:** 5

Ingredients:

- 2 cups spelt flakes
- 2 cups puffed cereal
- ¼ cup sunflower seeds
- ¼ cup almonds
- ¼ cup raisins
- ¼ cup dried cranberries
- ¼ cup chopped dried figs
- ¼ cup shredded coconut
- ¼ cup non-dairy chocolate chips
- 3 tsp ground cinnamon
- ½ cup coconut milk
- ½ cup blueberries

Directions:

❖ • In a bowl, combine the spelt flakes, puffed cereal, sunflower seeds, almonds, raisins, cranberries, figs, coconut, chocolate chips, and cinnamon. Toss to mix well. Pour in the coconut milk. Let sit for 1 hour and serve topped with blueberries

159) BERRY AND ALMOND BUTTER SWIRL BOWL

Preparation Time: 10 minutes **Servings:** 3

Ingredients:

- 1 ½ cups almond milk
- 2 small bananas
- 2 cups mixed berries, fresh or frozen
- 3 dates, pitted
- 3 scoops hemp protein powder
- 3 tbsp smooth almond butter
- 2 tbsp pepitas

Directions:

- In your blender or food processor, mix the almond milk with the bananas, berries and dates.
- Process until everything is well combined. Divide the smoothie between three bowls.
- Top each smoothie bowl with almond butter and use a butter knife to swirl the almond butter into the top of each smoothie bowl.
- Afterwards, garnish each smoothie bowl with pepitas, serve well-chilled and enjoy

160) OATS WITH COCONUT AND STRAWBERRIES

Preparation Time: 15 minutes **Servings:** 2

Ingredients:

- 1/2 tbsp coconut oil
- 1 cup rolled oats
- A pinch of flaky sea salt
- 1/8 tsp grated nutmeg
- 1/4 tsp cardamom
- 1 tbsp coconut sugar
- 1 cup coconut milk, sweetened
- 1 cup water
- 2 tbsp coconut flakes
- 4 tbsp fresh strawberries

Directions:

- In a saucepan, melt the coconut oil over a moderate flame. Then, toast the oats for about 3 minutes, stirring continuously.
- Add in the salt, nutmeg, cardamom, coconut sugar, milk and water; continue to cook for 12 minutes more or until cooked through.
- Spoon the mixture into serving bowls; top with coconut flakes and fresh strawberries. Enjoy

The Plant-Based for Athlete

SOUPS, STEW, AND SALADS

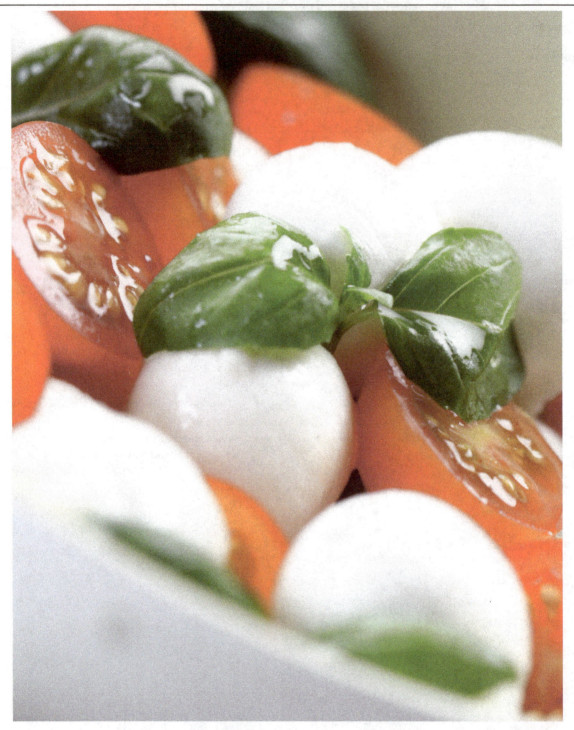

161) BLACK BEAN QUINOA SALAD

Preparation Time: 15 minutes + chilling time

Servings: 4

Ingredients:

- 2 cups water
- 1 cup quinoa, rinsed
- 16 ounces canned black beans, drained
- 2 Roma tomatoes, sliced
- 1 red onion, thinly sliced
- 1 cucumber, seeded and chopped
- 2 cloves garlic, pressed or minced
- 2 Italian peppers, seeded and sliced
- 2 tbsp fresh parsley, chopped
- 2 tbsp fresh cilantro, chopped
- 1/4 cup olive oil
- 1 lemon, freshly squeezed
- 1 tbsp apple cider vinegar
- 1/2 tsp dried dill weed
- 1/2 tsp dried oregano
- Sea salt and ground black pepper, to taste

Directions:

- Place the water and quinoa in a saucepan and bring it to a rolling boil. Immediately turn the heat to a simmer.
- Let it simmer for about 13 minutes until the quinoa has absorbed all of the water; fluff the quinoa with a fork and let it cool completely. Then, transfer the quinoa to a salad bowl.
- Add the remaining ingredients to the salad bowl and toss to combine well. Enjoy

162) POWER BULGUR SALAD WITH HERBS

Preparation Time: 20 minutes + chilling time

Servings: 4

Ingredients:

- 2 cups water
- 1 cup bulgur
- 12 ounces canned chickpeas, drained
- 1 Persian cucumber, thinly sliced
- 2 bell peppers, seeded and thinly sliced
- 1 jalapeno pepper, seeded and thinly sliced
- 2 Roma tomatoes, sliced
- 1 onion, thinly sliced
- 2 tbsp fresh basil, chopped
- 2 tbsp fresh parsley, chopped
- 2 tbsp fresh mint, chopped
- 2 tbsp fresh chives, chopped
- 4 tbsp olive oil
- 1 tbsp balsamic vinegar
- 1 tbsp lemon juice
- 1 tsp fresh garlic, pressed
- Sea salt and freshly ground black pepper, to taste
- 2 tbsp nutritional yeast
- 1/2 cup Kalamata olives, sliced

Directions:

- In a saucepan, bring the water and bulgur to a boil. Immediately turn the heat to a simmer and let it cook for about 20 minutes or until the bulgur is tender and water is almost absorbed. Fluff with a fork and spread on a large tray to let cool.
- Place the bulgur in a salad bowl followed by the chickpeas, cucumber, peppers, tomatoes, onion, basil, parsley, mint and chives.
- In a small mixing dish, whisk the olive oil, balsamic vinegar, lemon juice, garlic, salt and black pepper. Dress the salad and toss to combine.
- Sprinkle nutritional yeast over the top, garnish with olives and serve at room temperature. Enjoy

163) ORIGINAL ROASTED PEPPER SALAD

Preparation Time: 15 minutes + chilling time

Servings: 3

Ingredients:

- 6 bell peppers
- 3 tbsp extra-virgin olive oil
- 3 tsp red wine vinegar
- 3 garlic cloves, finely chopped
- 2 tbsp fresh parsley, chopped
- Sea salt and freshly cracked black pepper, to taste
- 1/2 tsp red pepper flakes
- 6 tbsp pine nuts, roughly chopped

Directions:

- Broil the peppers on a parchment-lined baking sheet for about 10 minutes, rotating the pan halfway through the cooking time, until they are charred on all sides.
- Then, cover the peppers with a plastic wrap to steam. Discard the skin, seeds and cores.
- Slice the peppers into strips and toss them with the remaining ingredients. Place in your refrigerator until ready to serve. Enjoy

164) WINTER HEARTY QUINOA SOUP

Preparation Time: 25 minutes

Servings: 4

Ingredients:

- 2 tbsp olive oil
- 1 onion, chopped
- 2 carrots, peeled and chopped
- 1 parsnip, chopped
- 1 celery stalk, chopped
- 1 cup yellow squash, chopped
- 4 garlic cloves, pressed or minced
- 4 cups roasted vegetable broth
- 2 medium tomatoes, crushed
- 1 cup quinoa
- Sea salt and ground black pepper, to taste
- 1 bay laurel
- 2 cup Swiss chard, tough ribs removed and torn into pieces
- 2 tbsp Italian parsley, chopped

Directions:

- In a heavy-bottomed pot, heat the olive over medium-high heat. Now, sauté the onion, carrot, parsnip, celery and yellow squash for about 3 minutes or until the vegetables are just tender.
- Add in the garlic and continue to sauté for 1 minute or until aromatic.
- Then, stir in the vegetable broth, tomatoes, quinoa, salt, pepper and bay laurel; bring to a boil. Immediately reduce the heat to a simmer and let it cook for 13 minutes.
- Fold in the Swiss chard; continue to simmer until the chard wilts.
- Ladle into individual bowls and serve garnished with the fresh parsley. Enjoy

165) GREEN LENTIL SALAD

Preparation Time: 20 minutes + chilling time

Servings: 5

Ingredients:

- 1 ½ cups green lentils, rinsed
- 2 cups arugula
- 2 cups Romaine lettuce, torn into pieces
- 1 cup baby spinach
- 1/4 cup fresh basil, chopped
- 1/2 cup shallots, chopped
- 2 garlic cloves, finely chopped
- 1/4 cup oil-packed sun-dried tomatoes, rinsed and chopped
- 5 tbsp extra-virgin olive oil
- 3 tbsp fresh lemon juice
- Sea salt and ground black pepper, to taste

Directions:

- In a large-sized saucepan, bring 4 ½ cups of the water and red lentils to a boil.
- Immediately turn the heat to a simmer and continue to cook your lentils for a further 15 to 17 minutes or until they've softened but not mushy. Drain and let it cool completely.
- Transfer the lentils to a salad bowl; toss the lentils with the remaining ingredients until well combined.
- Serve chilled or at room temperature. Enjoy

166) CHICKPEA, ACORN SQUASH, AND COUSCOUS SOUP

Preparation Time: 20 minutes

Servings: 4

Ingredients:

- 2 tbsp olive oil
- 1 shallot, chopped
- 1 carrot, trimmed and chopped
- 2 cups acorn squash, chopped
- 1 stalk celery, chopped
- 1 tsp garlic, finely chopped
- 1 tsp dried rosemary, chopped
- 1 tsp dried thyme, chopped
- 2 cups cream of onion soup
- 2 cups water
- 1 cup dry couscous
- Sea salt and ground black pepper, to taste
- 1/2 tsp red pepper flakes
- 6 ounces canned chickpeas, drained
- 2 tbsp fresh lemon juice

Directions:

- In a heavy-bottomed pot, heat the olive over medium-high heat. Now, sauté the shallot, carrot, acorn squash and celery for about 3 minutes or until the vegetables are just tender.
- Add in the garlic, rosemary and thyme and continue to sauté for 1 minute or until aromatic.
- Then, stir in the soup, water, couscous, salt, black pepper and red pepper flakes; bring to a boil. Immediately reduce the heat to a simmer and let it cook for 12 minutes.
- Fold in the canned chickpeas; continue to simmer until heated through or about 5 minutes more.
- Ladle into individual bowls and drizzle with the lemon juice over the top. Enjoy

167) GARLIC CROSTINI WITH CABBAGE SOUP

Preparation Time: 1 hour **Servings:** 4

Ingredients:

- Soup:
- 2 tbsp olive oil
- 1 medium leek, chopped
- 1 cup turnip, chopped
- 1 parsnip, chopped
- 1 carrot, chopped
- 2 cups cabbage, shredded
- 2 garlic cloves, finely chopped
- 4 cups vegetable broth
- 2 bay leaves
- Sea salt and ground black pepper, to taste
- 1/4 tsp cumin seeds
- 1/2 tsp mustard seeds
- 1 tsp dried basil
- 2 tomatoes, pureed
- Crostini:
- 8 slices of baguette
- 2 heads garlic
- 4 tbsp extra-virgin olive oil

Directions:

- In a soup pot, heat 2 tbsp of the olive over medium-high heat. Now, sauté the leek, turnip, parsnip and carrot for about 4 minutes or until the vegetables are crisp-tender.
- Add in the garlic and cabbage and continue to sauté for 1 minute or until aromatic.
- Then, stir in the vegetable broth, bay leaves, salt, black pepper, cumin seeds, mustard seeds, dried basil and pureed tomatoes; bring to a boil. Immediately reduce the heat to a simmer and let it cook for about 20 minutes.
- Meanwhile, preheat your oven to 375 degrees F. Now, roast the garlic and baguette slices for about 15 minutes. Remove the crostini from the oven.
- Continue baking the garlic for 45 minutes more or until very tender. Allow the garlic to cool.
- Now, cut each head of the garlic using a sharp serrated knife in order to separate all the cloves.
- Squeeze the roasted garlic cloves out of their skins. Mash the garlic pulp with 4 tbsp of the extra-virgin olive oil.
- Spread the roasted garlic mixture evenly on the tops of the crostini. Serve with the warm soup. Enjoy

168) GREEN BEAN SOUP CREAM

Preparation Time: 35 minutes **Servings:** 4

Ingredients:

- 1 tbsp sesame oil
- 1 onion, chopped
- 1 green pepper, seeded and chopped
- 2 russet potatoes, peeled and diced
- 2 garlic cloves, chopped
- 4 cups vegetable broth
- 1 pound green beans, trimmed
- Sea salt and ground black pepper, to season
- 1 cup full-fat coconut milk

Directions:

- In a heavy-bottomed pot, heat the sesame over medium-high heat. Now, sauté the onion, peppers and potatoes for about 5 minutes, stirring periodically. Add in the garlic and continue sautéing for 1 minute or until fragrant.
- Then, stir in the vegetable broth, green beans, salt and black pepper; bring to a boil. Immediately reduce the heat to a simmer and let it cook for 20 minutes.
- Puree the green bean mixture using an immersion blender until creamy and uniform.
- Return the pureed mixture to the pot. Fold in the coconut milk and continue to simmer until heated through or about 5 minutes longer.
- Ladle into individual bowls and serve hot. Enjoy

The Plant-Based for Athlete

169) FRENCH TRADITIONAL ONION SOUP

Preparation Time: 1 hour 30 minutes

Servings: 4

Ingredients:

- 2 tbsp olive oil
- 2 large yellow onions, thinly sliced
- 2 thyme sprigs, chopped
- 2 rosemary sprigs, chopped
- 2 tsp balsamic vinegar
- 4 cups vegetable stock
- Sea salt and ground black pepper, to taste

Directions:

- In a or Dutch oven, heat the olive oil over a moderate heat. Now, cook the onions with thyme, rosemary and 1 tsp of the sea salt for about 2 minutes.
- Now, turn the heat to medium-low and continue cooking until the onions caramelize or about 50 minutes.
- Add in the balsamic vinegar and continue to cook for a further 15 more. Add in the stock, salt and black pepper and continue simmering for 20 to 25 minutes.
- Serve with toasted bread and enjoy

170) ROASTED CARROT SOUP

Preparation Time: 50 minutes

Servings: 4

Ingredients:

- 1 ½ pounds carrots
- 4 tbsp olive oil
- 1 yellow onion, chopped
- 2 cloves garlic, minced
- 1/3 tsp ground cumin
- Sea salt and white pepper, to taste
- 1/2 tsp turmeric powder
- 4 cups vegetable stock
- 2 tsp lemon juice
- 2 tbsp fresh cilantro, roughly chopped

Directions:

- Start by preheating your oven to 400 degrees F. Place the carrots on a large parchment-lined baking sheet; toss the carrots with 2 tbsp of the olive oil.
- Roast the carrots for about 35 minutes or until they've softened.
- In a heavy-bottomed pot, heat the remaining 2 tbsp of the olive oil. Now, sauté the onion and garlic for about 3 minutes or until aromatic.
- Add in the cumin, salt, pepper, turmeric, vegetable stock and roasted carrots. Continue to simmer for 12 minutes more.
- Puree your soup with an immersion blender. Drizzle lemon juice over your soup and serve garnished with fresh cilantro leaves. Enjoy

171) ITALIAN PENNE PASTA SALAD

Preparation Time: 15 minutes + chilling time

Servings: 3

Ingredients:

- 9 ounces penne pasta
- 9 ounces canned Cannellini bean, drained
- 1 small onion, thinly sliced
- 1/3 cup Niçoise olives, pitted and sliced
- 2 Italian peppers, sliced
- 1 cup cherry tomatoes, halved
- 3 cups arugula

- Dressing:
- 3 tbsp extra-virgin olive oil
- 1 tsp lemon zest
- 1 tsp garlic, minced
- 3 tbsp balsamic vinegar
- 1 tsp Italian herb mix
- Sea salt and ground black pepper, to taste

Directions:

- Cook the penne pasta according to the package directions. Drain and rinse the pasta. Let it cool completely and then, transfer it to a salad bowl.
- Then, add the beans, onion, olives, peppers, tomatoes and arugula to the salad bowl.
- Mix all the dressing ingredients until everything is well incorporated. Dress your salad and serve well

172) CHANA CHAAT INDIAN SALAD

Preparation Time: 45 minutes + chilling time

Servings: 4

Ingredients:

- 1 pound dry chickpeas, soaked overnight
- 2 San Marzano tomatoes, diced
- 1 Persian cucumber, sliced
- 1 onion, chopped
- 1 bell pepper, seeded and thinly sliced
- 1 green chili, seeded and thinly sliced
- 2 handfuls baby spinach
- 1/2 tsp Kashmiri chili powder

- 4 curry leaves, chopped
- 1 tbsp chaat masala
- 2 tbsp fresh lemon juice, or to taste
- 4 tbsp olive oil
- 1 tsp agave syrup
- 1/2 tsp mustard seeds
- 1/2 tsp coriander seeds
- 2 tbsp sesame seeds, lightly toasted
- 2 tbsp fresh cilantro, roughly chopped

Directions:

- Drain the chickpeas and transfer them to a large saucepan. Cover the chickpeas with water by 2 inches and bring it to a boil.
- Immediately turn the heat to a simmer and continue to cook for approximately 40 minutes.
- Toss the chickpeas with the tomatoes, cucumber, onion, peppers, spinach, chili powder, curry leaves and chaat masala.
- In a small mixing dish, thoroughly combine the lemon juice, olive oil, agave syrup, mustard seeds and coriander seeds.
- Garnish with sesame seeds and fresh cilantro. Enjoy

173) TEMPEH AND NOODLE SALAD THAI-STYLE

Preparation Time: 45 minutes **Servings:** 3

Ingredients:

- 6 ounces tempeh
- 4 tbsp rice vinegar
- 4 tbsp soy sauce
- 2 garlic cloves, minced
- 1 small-sized lime, freshly juiced
- 5 ounces rice noodles
- 1 carrot, julienned
- 1 shallot, chopped
- 3 handfuls Chinese cabbage, thinly sliced
- 3 handfuls kale, torn into pieces
- 1 bell pepper, seeded and thinly sliced
- 1 bird's eye chili, minced
- 1/4 cup peanut butter
- 2 tbsp agave syrup

Directions:

- Place the tempeh, 2 tbsp of the rice vinegar, soy sauce, garlic and lime juice in a ceramic dish; let it marinate for about 40 minutes.
- Meanwhile, cook the rice noodles according to the package directions. Drain your noodles and transfer them to a salad bowl.
- Add the carrot, shallot, cabbage, kale and peppers to the salad bowl. Add in the peanut butter, the remaining 2 tbsp of the rice vinegar and agave syrup and toss to combine well.
- Top with the marinated tempeh and serve immediately. Enjoy

174) TYPICAL CREAM OF BROCCOLI SOUP

Preparation Time: 35 minutes **Servings:** 4

Ingredients:

- 2 tbsp olive oil
- 1 pound broccoli florets
- 1 onion, chopped
- 1 celery rib, chopped
- 1 parsnip, chopped
- 1 tsp garlic, chopped
- 3 cups vegetable broth
- 1/2 tsp dried dill
- 1/2 tsp dried oregano
- Sea salt and ground black pepper, to taste
- 2 tbsp flaxseed meal
- 1 cup full-fat coconut milk

Directions:

- In a heavy-bottomed pot, heat the olive oil over medium-high heat. Now, sauté the broccoli onion, celery and parsnip for about 5 minutes, stirring periodically.
- Add in the garlic and continue sautéing for 1 minute or until fragrant.
- Then, stir in the vegetable broth, dill, oregano, salt and black pepper; bring to a boil. Immediately reduce the heat to a simmer and let it cook for about 20 minutes.
- Puree the soup using an immersion blender until creamy and uniform.
- Return the pureed mixture to the pot. Fold in the flaxseed meal and coconut milk; continue to simmer until heated through or about 5 minutes.
- Ladle into four serving bowls and enjoy

175) RAISIN MOROCCAN LENTIL SALAD

Preparation Time: 20 minutes + chilling time

Servings: 4

Ingredients:

- 1 cup red lentils, rinsed
- 1 large carrot, julienned
- 1 Persian cucumber, thinly sliced
- 1 sweet onion, chopped
- 1/2 cup golden raisins
- 1/4 cup fresh mint, snipped
- 1/4 cup fresh basil, snipped
- 1/4 cup extra-virgin olive oil
- 1/4 cup lemon juice, freshly squeezed
- 1 tsp grated lemon peel
- 1/2 tsp fresh ginger root, peeled and minced
- 1/2 tsp granulated garlic
- 1 tsp ground allspice
- Sea salt and ground black pepper, to taste

Directions:

- In a large-sized saucepan, bring 3 cups of the water and 1 cup of the lentils to a boil.
- Immediately turn the heat to a simmer and continue to cook your lentils for a further 15 to 17 minutes or until they've softened but are not mushy yet. Drain and let it cool completely.
- Transfer the lentils to a salad bowl; add in the carrot, cucumber and sweet onion. Then, add the raisins, mint and basil to your salad.
- In a small mixing dish, whisk the olive oil, lemon juice, lemon peel, ginger, granulated garlic, allspice, salt and black pepper.
- Dress your salad and serve well-chilled. Enjoy

176) CHICKPEA AND ASPARAGUS SALAD

Preparation Time: 10 minutes + chilling time

Servings: 5

Ingredients:

- 1 ¼ pounds asparagus, trimmed and cut into bite-sized pieces
- 5 ounces canned chickpeas, drained and rinsed
- 1 chipotle pepper, seeded and chopped
- 1 Italian pepper, seeded and chopped
- 1/4 cup fresh basil leaves, chopped
- 1/4 cup fresh parsley leaves, chopped
- 2 tbsp fresh mint leaves
- 2 tbsp fresh chives, chopped
- 1 tsp garlic, minced
- 1/4 cup extra-virgin olive oil
- 1 tbsp balsamic vinegar
- 1 tbsp fresh lime juice
- 2 tbsp soy sauce
- 1/4 tsp ground allspice
- 1/4 tsp ground cumin
- Sea salt and freshly cracked peppercorns, to taste

Directions:

- Bring a large pot of salted water with the asparagus to a boil; let it cook for 2 minutes; drain and rinse.
- Transfer the asparagus to a salad bowl.
- Toss the asparagus with the chickpeas, peppers, herbs, garlic, olive oil, vinegar, lime juice, soy sauce and spices.
- Toss to combine and serve immediately. Enjoy

177) QUINOA AND AVOCADO SALAD

Preparation Time: 15 minutes + chilling time

Servings: 4

Ingredients:

- 1 cup quinoa, rinsed
- 1 onion, chopped
- 1 tomato, diced
- 2 roasted peppers, cut into strips
- 2 tbsp parsley, chopped
- 2 tbsp basil, chopped
- 1/4 cup extra-virgin olive oil
- 2 tbsp red wine vinegar
- 2 tbsp lemon juice
- 1/4 tsp cayenne pepper
- Sea salt and freshly ground black pepper, to season
- 1 avocado, peeled, pitted and sliced
- 1 tbsp sesame seeds, toasted

Directions:

- Place the water and quinoa in a saucepan and bring it to a rolling boil. Immediately turn the heat to a simmer.
- Let it simmer for about 13 minutes until the quinoa has absorbed all of the water; fluff the quinoa with a fork and let it cool completely. Then, transfer the quinoa to a salad bowl.
- Add the onion, tomato, roasted peppers, parsley and basil to the salad bowl. In another small bowl, whisk the olive oil, vinegar, lemon juice, cayenne pepper, salt and black pepper.
- Dress your salad and toss to combine well. Top with avocado slices and garnish with toasted sesame seeds.
- Enjoy

178) TABBOULEH SALAD WITH TOFU

Preparation Time: 20 minutes + chilling time

Servings: 4

Ingredients:

- 1 cup bulgur wheat
- 2 San Marzano tomatoes, sliced
- 1 Persian cucumber, thinly sliced
- 2 tbsp basil, chopped
- 2 tbsp parsley, chopped
- 4 scallions, chopped
- 2 cups arugula
- 2 cups baby spinach, torn into pieces
- 4 tbsp tahini
- 4 tbsp lemon juice
- 1 tbsp soy sauce
- 1 tsp fresh garlic, pressed
- Sea salt and ground black pepper, to taste
- 12 ounces smoked tofu, cubed

Directions:

- In a saucepan, bring 2 cups of water and the bulgur to a boil. Immediately turn the heat to a simmer and let it cook for about 20 minutes or until the bulgur is tender and the water is almost absorbed. Fluff with a fork and spread on a large tray to let cool.
- Place the bulgur in a salad bowl followed by the tomatoes, cucumber, basil, parsley, scallions, arugula and spinach.
- In a small mixing dish, whisk the tahini, lemon juice, soy sauce, garlic, salt and black pepper. Dress the salad and toss to combine.
- Top your salad with the smoked tofu and serve at room temperature. Enjoy

179) GREEN PASTA SALAD

Preparation Time: 10 minutes + chilling time

Servings: 4

Ingredients:

- 12 ounces rotini pasta
- 1 small onion, thinly sliced
- 1 cup cherry tomatoes, halved
- 1 bell pepper, chopped
- 1 jalapeno pepper, chopped
- 1 tbsp capers, drained
- 2 cups Iceberg lettuce, torn into pieces
- 2 tbsp fresh parsley, chopped
- 2 tbsp fresh cilantro, chopped
- 2 tbsp fresh basil, chopped
- 1/4 cup olive oil
- 2 tbsp apple cider vinegar
- 1 tsp garlic, pressed
- Kosher salt and ground black pepper, to taste
- 2 tbsp nutritional yeast
- 2 tbsp pine nuts, toasted and chopped

Directions:

- Cook the pasta according to the package directions. Drain and rinse the pasta. Let it cool completely and then, transfer it to a salad bowl.
- Then, add in the onion, tomatoes, peppers, capers, lettuce, parsley, cilantro and basil to the salad bowl.
- Whisk the olive oil, vinegar, garlic, salt, black pepper and nutritional yeast. Dress your salad and top with toasted pine nuts. Enjoy

180) ORIGINAL UKRAINIAN BORSCHT

Preparation Time: 40 minutes

Servings: 4

Ingredients:

- 2 tbsp sesame oil
- 1 red onion, chopped
- 2 carrots, trimmed and sliced
- 2 large beets, peeled and sliced
- 2 large potatoes, peeled and diced
- 4 cups vegetable stock
- 2 garlic cloves, minced
- 1/2 tsp caraway seeds
- 1/2 tsp celery seeds
- 1/2 tsp fennel seeds
- 1 pound red cabbage, shredded
- 1/2 tsp mixed peppercorns, freshly cracked
- Kosher salt, to taste
- 2 bay leaves
- 2 tbsp wine vinegar

Directions:

- In a Dutch oven, heat the sesame oil over a moderate flame. Once hot, sauté the onions until tender and translucent, about 6 minutes.
- Add in the carrots, beets and potatoes and continue to sauté an additional 10 minutes, adding the vegetable stock periodically.
- Next, stir in the garlic, caraway seeds, celery seeds, fennel seeds and continue sautéing for another 30 seconds.
- Add in the cabbage, mixed peppercorns, salt and bay leaves. Add in the remaining stock and bring to boil.
- Immediately turn the heat to a simmer and continue to cook for 20 to 23 minutes longer until the vegetables have softened.
- Ladle into individual bowls and drizzle wine vinegar over it. Serve and enjoy

181) LENTIL BELUGA SALAD

Preparation Time: 20 minutes + chilling time

Servings: 4

Ingredients:

- 1 cup Beluga lentils, rinsed
- 1 Persian cucumber, sliced
- 1 large-sized tomatoes, sliced
- 1 red onion, chopped
- 1 bell pepper, sliced
- 1/4 cup fresh basil, chopped
- 1/4 cup fresh Italian parsley, chopped
- 2 ounces green olives, pitted and sliced
- 1/4 cup olive oil
- 4 tbsp lemon juice
- 1 tsp deli mustard
- 1/2 tsp garlic, minced
- 1/2 tsp red pepper flakes, crushed
- Sea salt and ground black pepper, to taste

Directions:

- In a large-sized saucepan, bring 3 cups of the water and 1 cup of the lentils to a boil.
- Immediately turn the heat to a simmer and continue to cook your lentils for a further 15 to 17 minutes or until they've softened but not mushy. Drain and let it cool completely.
- Transfer the lentils to a salad bowl; add in the cucumber, tomatoes, onion, pepper, basil, parsley and olives.
- In a small mixing dish, whisk the olive oil, lemon juice, mustard, garlic, red pepper, salt and black pepper.
- Dress the salad, toss to combine and serve well-chilled. Enjoy

182) INDIAN NAAN SALAD

Preparation Time: 10 minutes

Servings: 3

Ingredients:

- 3 tbsp sesame oil
- 1 tsp ginger, peeled and minced
- 1/2 tsp cumin seeds
- 1/2 tsp mustard seeds
- 1/2 tsp mixed peppercorns
- 1 tbsp curry leaves
- 3 naan breads, broken into bite-sized pieces
- 1 shallot, chopped
- 2 tomatoes, chopped
- Himalayan salt, to taste
- 1 tbsp soy sauce

Directions:

- Heat 2 tbsp of the sesame oil in a non-stick skillet over a moderately high heat.
- Sauté the ginger, cumin seeds, mustard seeds, mixed peppercorns and curry leaves for 1 minute or so, until fragrant.
- Stir in the naan breads and continue to cook, stirring periodically, until golden-brown and well coated with the spices.
- Place the shallot and tomatoes in a salad bowl; toss them with the salt, soy sauce and the remaining 1 tbsp of the sesame oil.
- Place the toasted naan on the top of your salad and serve at room temperature. Enjoy

183) BROCCOLI GINGER SOUP

Preparation Time: 50 minutes

Servings: 4

Ingredients:

- 1 onion, chopped
- 1 tbsp minced peeled fresh ginger
- 2 tsp olive oil
- 2 carrots, chopped
- 1 head broccoli, chopped into florets
- 1 cup coconut milk
- 3 cups vegetable broth
- ½ tsp turmeric
- Salt and black pepper to taste

Directions:

- In a pot over medium heat, place the onion, ginger, and olive oil, cook for 4 minutes. Add in carrots, broccoli, broth, turmeric, pepper, and salt. Bring to a boil and cook for 15 minutes. Transfer the soup to a food processor and blend until smooth. Stir in coconut milk and serve warm

184) NOODLE RICE SOUP WITH BEANS

Preparation Time: 10 minutes

Servings: 6

Ingredients:

- 2 carrots, chopped
- 2 celery stalks, chopped
- 6 cups vegetable broth
- 8 oz brown rice noodles
- 1 (15-oz) can pinto beans
- 1 tsp dried herbs

Directions:

- Place a pot over medium heat and add in the carrots, celery, and vegetable broth. Bring to a boil. Add in noodles, beans, dried herbs, salt, and pepper. Reduce the heat and simmer for 5 minutes. Serve

185) VEGETABLE AND RICE SOUP

Preparation Time: 40 minutes

Servings: 6

Ingredients:

- 3 tbsp olive oil
- 2 carrots, chopped
- 1 onion, chopped
- 1 celery stalk, chopped
- 2 garlic cloves, minced
- 2 cups chopped cabbage
- ½ red bell pepper, chopped
- 4 potatoes, unpeeled and quartered
- 6 cups vegetable broth
- ½ cup brown rice, rinsed
- ½ cup frozen green peas
- 2 tbsp chopped parsley

Directions:

- Heat the oil in a pot over medium heat. Place carrots, onion, celery, and garlic. Cook for 5 minutes. Add in cabbage, bell pepper, potatoes, and broth. Bring to a boil, then lower the heat and add the brown rice, salt, and pepper. Simmer uncovered for 25 minutes until vegetables are tender. Stir in peas and cook for 5 minutes. Top with parsley and serve warm

186) DAIKON AND SWEET POTATO SOUP

Preparation Time: 40 minutes

Servings: 6

Ingredients:

- 6 cups water
- 2 tsp olive oil
- 1 chopped onion
- 3 garlic cloves, minced
- 1 tbsp thyme
- 2 tsp paprika
- 2 cups peeled and chopped daikon
- 2 cups chopped sweet potatoes
- 2 cups peeled and chopped parsnips
- ½ tsp sea salt
- 1 cup fresh mint, chopped
- ½ avocado
- 2 tbsp balsamic vinegar
- 2 tbsp pumpkin seeds

Directions:

- Heat the oil in a pot and place onion and garlic. Sauté for 3 minutes. Add in thyme, paprika, daikon, sweet potato, parsnips, water, and salt. Bring to a boil and cook for 30 minutes. Remove the soup to a food processor and add in balsamic vinegar; purée until smooth. Top with mint and pumpkin seeds to serve

187) CHICKPEA AND VEGETABLE SOUP

Preparation Time: 35 minutes

Servings: 5

Ingredients:

- 2 tbsp olive oil
- 1 onion, chopped
- 1 carrot, chopped
- 1 celery stalk, chopped
- 2 tsp smoked paprika
- 1 tsp ground cumin
- 1 tsp za'atar spice
- ¼ tsp ground cayenne pepper
- 6 cups vegetable

Directions:

- Heat the oil in a pot over medium heat. Place onion, carrot, and celery and cook for 5 minutes. Add in eggplant, tomatoes, tomato paste, chickpeas, paprika, cumin, za´atar spice, and cayenne pepper. Stir in broth and salt. Bring to a

- 1 eggplant, chopped
- 1 (28-oz) can diced tomatoes
- 2 tbsp tomato paste
- 1 (15.5-oz) can chickpeas, drained
- broth
- 4 oz whole-wheat vermicelli
- 2 tbsp minced cilantro

boil, then lower the heat and simmer for 15 minutes. Add in vermicelli and cook for another 5 minutes. Serve topped with cilantro

188) ITALIAN-STYLE BEAN SOUP

Preparation Time: 1 hour 25 minutes

Servings: 6

Ingredients:
- 3 tbsp olive oil
- 2 celery stalks, chopped
- 2 carrots, chopped
- 3 shallots, chopped
- 3 garlic cloves, minced
- ½ cup brown rice
- 6 cups vegetable broth
- 1 (14.5-oz) can diced tomatoes
- 2 bay leaves
- Salt and black pepper to taste
- 2 (15.5-oz) cans white beans
- ¼ cup chopped basil

Directions:
- Heat oil in a pot over medium heat. Place celery, carrots, shallots, and garlic and cook for 5 minutes. Add in brown rice, broth, tomatoes, bay leaves, salt, and pepper. Bring to a boil, then lower the heat and simmer uncovered for 20 minutes. Stir in beans and basil and cook for 5 minutes. Discard bay leaves and spoon into bowls. Sprinkle with basil and serve

189) BRUSSELS SPROUTS AND TOFU SOUP

Preparation Time: 40 minutes

Servings: 4

Ingredients:
- 7 oz firm tofu, cubed
- 2 tsp olive oil
- 1 cup sliced mushrooms
- 1 cup shredded Brussels sprouts
- 1 garlic clove, minced
- ½-inch piece fresh ginger, minced
- Salt to taste
- 2 tbsp apple cider vinegar
- 2 tbsp soy sauce
- 1 tsp pure date sugar
- ¼ tsp red pepper flakes
- 1 scallion, chopped

Directions:
- Heat the oil in a skillet over medium heat. Place mushrooms, Brussels sprouts, garlic, ginger, and salt. Sauté for 7-8 minutes until the veggies are soft. Pour in 4 cups of water, vinegar, soy sauce, sugar, pepper flakes, and tofu. Bring to a boil, then lower the heat and simmer for 5-10 minutes. Top with scallions and serve

190) WHITE BEAN ROSEMARY SOUP

Preparation Time: 30 minutes

Servings: 4

Ingredients:
- 2 tsp olive oil
- 1 carrot, chopped
- 1 onion, chopped
- 2 garlic cloves, minced
- 1 tbsp rosemary, chopped
- 2 tbsp apple cider vinegar
- 1 cup dried white beans
- ¼ tsp salt
- 2 tbsp nutritional yeast

Directions:
- Heat the oil in a pot over medium heat. Place carrots, onion, and garlic and cook for 5 minutes.
- Pour in vinegar to deglaze the pot. Stir in 5 cups water and beans and bring to a boil. Lower the heat and simmer for 45 minutes until the beans are soft. Add in salt and nutritional yeast and stir. Serve topped with chopped rosemary

The Plant-Based for Athlete

191) MUSHROOM AND TOFU SOUP

Preparation Time: 20 minutes

Servings: 4

Ingredients:

- 4 cups water
- 2 tbsp soy sauce
- 4 white mushrooms, sliced
- ¼ cup chopped green onions
- 3 tbsp tahini
- 6 oz extra-firm tofu, diced

Directions:

- Pour the water and soy sauce into a pot and bring to a boil. Add in mushrooms and green onions. Lower the heat and simmer for 10 minutes. In a bowl, combine ½ cup of hot soup with tahini. Pour the mixture into the pot and simmer 2 minutes more, but not boil. Stir in tofu. Serve warm

192) AUTUMN ROOT VEGETABLE SOUP

Preparation Time: 40 minutes

Servings: 4

Ingredients:

- 4 tbsp avocado oil
- 1 large leek, sliced
- 2 carrots, diced
- 2 parsnips, diced
- 2 cups turnip, diced
- 2 celery stalks, diced
- 1 pound sweet potatoes, diced
- 1 tsp ginger-garlic paste
- 1 habanero pepper, seeded and chopped
- 1/2 tsp caraway seeds
- 1/2 tsp fennel seeds
- 2 bay leaves
- Sea salt and ground black pepper, to season
- 1 tsp cayenne pepper
- 4 cups vegetable broth
- 4 tbsp tahini

Directions:

- In a stockpot, heat the oil over medium-high heat. Now, sauté the leeks, carrots, parsnip, turnip, celery and sweet potatoes for about 5 minutes, stirring periodically.
- Add in the ginger-garlic paste and habanero peppers and continue sautéing for 1 minute or until fragrant.
- Then, stir in the caraway seeds, fennel seeds, bay leaves, salt, black pepper, cayenne pepper and vegetable broth; bring to a boil. Immediately turn the heat to a simmer and let it cook for approximately 25 minutes.
- Puree the soup using an immersion blender until creamy and uniform.
- Return the pureed mixture to the pot. Fold in the tahini and continue to simmer until heated through or about 5 minutes longer.
- Ladle into individual bowls and serve hot. Enjoy

193) GREEK SALAD

Preparation Time: 10 minutes

Servings: 2

Ingredients:

- ½ yellow bell pepper, cut into pieces
- 3 tomatoes cut into bite-size pieces
- ½ cucumber, cut into
- ½ cup tofu cheese, cut into squares
- 10 Kalamata olives, pitted
- ½ tbsp red wine vinegar
- 4 tbsp olive oil

Directions:

- Pour the bell pepper, tomatoes, cucumber, red onion, tofu cheese, and olives into a salad bowl. Drizzle the red wine vinegar and olive oil over the vegetables. Season with salt, black pepper, and oregano, and toss the salad with two spoons. Share

- bite-size pieces
- ½ red onion, peeled and sliced
- 2 tsp dried oregano

the salad into two bowls and serve immediately

The Plant-Based for Athlete

VEGETABLES AND SIDE DISHES

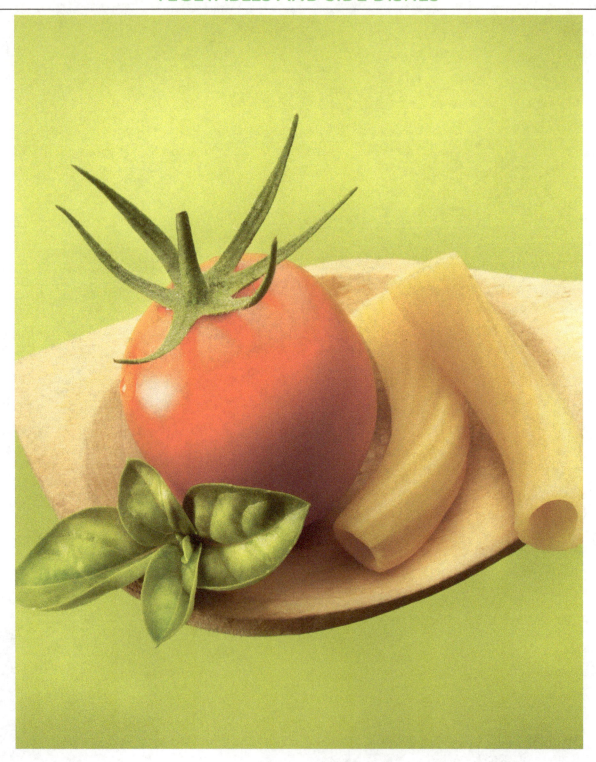

194) CHINESE CABBAGE STIR-FRY

Preparation Time: 10 minutes

Servings: 3

Ingredients:

- 3 tbsp sesame oil
- 1 pound Chinese cabbage, sliced
- 1/2 tsp Chinese five-spice powder
- Kosher salt, to taste
- 1/2 tsp Szechuan pepper
- 2 tbsp soy sauce
- 3 tbsp sesame seeds, lightly toasted

Directions:

- In a wok, heat the sesame oil until sizzling. Stir fry the cabbage for about 5 minutes.
- Stir in the spices and soy sauce and continue to cook, stirring frequently, for about 5 minutes more, until the cabbage is crisp-tender and aromatic.
- Sprinkle sesame seeds over the top and serve immediately

195) SAUTÉED CAULIFLOWER WITH SESAME SEEDS

Preparation Time: 15 minutes

Servings: 4

Ingredients:

- 1 cup vegetable broth
- 1 ½ pounds cauliflower florets
- 4 tbsp olive oil
- 2 scallion stalks, chopped
- 4 garlic cloves, minced
- Sea salt and freshly ground black pepper, to taste
- 2 tbsp sesame seeds, lightly toasted

Directions:

- In a large saucepan, bring the vegetable broth to a boil; then, add in the cauliflower and cook for about 6 minutes or until fork-tender; reserve.
- Then, heat the olive oil until sizzling; now, sauté the scallions and garlic for about 1 minute or until tender and aromatic.
- Add in the reserved cauliflower, followed by salt and black pepper; continue to simmer for about 5 minutes or until heated through
- Garnish with toasted sesame seeds and serve immediately. Enjoy

196) SWEET MASHED CARROTS

Preparation Time: 25 minutes

Servings: 4

Ingredients:

- 1 ½ pounds carrots, trimmed
- 3 tbsp vegan butter
- 1 cup scallions, sliced
- 1 tbsp maple syrup
- 1/2 tsp garlic powder
- 1/2 tsp ground allspice
- Sea salt, to taste
- 1/2 cup soy sauce
- 2 tbsp fresh cilantro, chopped

Directions:

- Steam the carrots for about 15 minutes until they are very tender; drain well.
- In a sauté pan, melt the butter until sizzling. Now, turn the heat down to maintain an insistent sizzle.
- Now, cook the scallions until they've softened. Add in the maple syrup, garlic powder, ground allspice, salt and soy sauce for about 10 minutes or until they are caramelized.
- Add the caramelized scallions to your food processor; add in the carrots and puree the ingredients until everything is well blended.
- Serve garnished with the fresh cilantro. Enjoy

197) SAUTÉED TURNIP GREENS

Preparation Time: 15 minutes

Servings: 4

Ingredients:

- 2 tbsp olive oil
- 1 onion, sliced
- 2 garlic cloves, sliced
- 1 ½ pounds turnip greens cleaned and chopped
- 1/4 cup vegetable broth
- 1/4 cup dry white wine
- 1/2 tsp dried oregano
- 1 tsp dried parsley flakes
- Kosher salt and ground black pepper, to taste

Directions:

- In a sauté pan, heat the olive oil over a moderately high heat.
- Now, sauté the onion for 3 to 4 minutes or until tender and translucent. Add in the garlic and continue to cook for 30 seconds more or until aromatic.
- Stir in the turnip greens, broth, wine, oregano and parsley; continue sautéing an additional 6 minutes or until they have wilted completely.
- Season with salt and black pepper to taste and serve warm. Enjoy

198) YUKON GOLD MASHED POTATOES

Preparation Time: 25 minutes

Servings: 5

Ingredients:

- 2 pounds Yukon Gold potatoes, peeled and diced
- 1 clove garlic, pressed
- Sea salt and red pepper flakes, to taste
- 3 tbsp vegan butter
- 1/2 cup soy milk
- 2 tbsp scallions, sliced

Directions:

- Cover the potatoes with an inch or two of cold water. Cook the potatoes in gently boiling water for about 20 minutes.
- Then, puree the potatoes, along with the garlic, salt, red pepper, butter and milk, to your desired consistency.
- Serve garnished with fresh scallions. Enjoy

199) AROMATIC SAUTÉED SWISS CHARD

Preparation Time: 15 minutes

Servings: 4

Ingredients:

- 2 tbsp vegan butter
- 1 onion, chopped
- 2 cloves garlic, sliced
- Sea salt and ground black pepper, to season
- 1 ½ pounds Swiss chard, torn into pieces, tough stalks removed
- 1 cup vegetable broth
- 1 bay leaf
- 1 thyme sprig
- 2 rosemary sprigs
- 1/2 tsp mustard seeds
- 1 tsp celery seeds

Directions:

- In a saucepan, melt the vegan butter over medium-high heat.
- Then, sauté the onion for about 3 minutes or until tender and translucent; sauté the garlic for about 1 minute until aromatic.
- Add in the remaining ingredients and turn the heat to a simmer; let it simmer, covered, for about 10 minutes or until everything is cooked through. Enjoy

200) CLASSIC SAUTÉED BELL PEPPERS

Preparation Time: 15 minutes

Servings: 2

Ingredients:

- 3 tbsp olive oil
- 4 bell peppers, seeded and slice into strips
- 2 cloves garlic, minced
- Salt and freshly ground black pepper, to taste
- 1 tsp cayenne pepper
- 4 tbsp dry white wine
- 2 tbsp fresh cilantro, roughly chopped

Directions:

- In a saucepan, heat the oil over medium-high heat.
- Once hot, sauté the peppers for about 4 minutes or until tender and fragrant. Then, sauté the garlic for about 1 minute until aromatic.
- Add in the salt, black pepper and cayenne pepper; continue to sauté, adding the wine, for about 6 minutes more until tender and cooked through.
- Taste and adjust the seasonings. Top with fresh cilantro and serve. Enjoy

201) MASHED ROOT VEGETABLES

Preparation Time: 25 minutes

Servings: 5

Ingredients:

- 1 pound russet potatoes, peeled and cut into chunks
- 1/2 pound parsnips, trimmed and diced
- 1/2 pound carrots, trimmed and diced
- 4 tbsp vegan butter
- 1 tsp dried oregano
- 1/2 tsp dried dill weed
- 1/2 tsp dried marjoram
- 1 tsp dried basil

Directions:

- Cover the vegetables with the water by 1 inch. Bring to a boil and cook for about 25 minutes until they've softened; drain.
- Mash the vegetables with the remaining ingredients, adding cooking liquid, as needed.
- Serve warm and enjoy

202) ROASTED BUTTERNUT SQUASH

Preparation Time: 25 minutes

Servings: 4

Ingredients:

- 4 tbsp olive oil
- 1/2 tsp ground cumin
- 1/2 tsp ground allspice
- 1 ½ pounds butternut squash, peeled, seeded and diced
- 1/4 cup dry white wine
- 2 tbsp dark soy sauce
- 1 tsp mustard seeds
- 1 tsp paprika
- Sea salt and ground black pepper, to taste

Directions:

- Start by preheating your oven to 420 degrees F. Toss the squash with the remaining ingredients.
- Roast the butternut squash for about 25 minutes or until tender and caramelized.
- Serve warm and enjoy

203) SAUTÉED CREMINI MUSHROOMS

Preparation Time: 10 minutes

Servings: 4

Ingredients:

- 4 tbsp olive oil
- 4 tbsp shallots, chopped
- 2 cloves garlic, minced
- 1 ½ pounds Cremini mushrooms, sliced
- 1/4 cup dry white wine
- Sea salt and ground black pepper, to taste

Directions:

- In a sauté pan, heat the olive oil over a moderately high heat.
- Now, sauté the shallot for 3 to 4 minutes or until tender and translucent. Add in the garlic and continue to cook for 30 seconds more or until aromatic.
- Stir in the Cremini mushrooms, wine, salt and black pepper; continue sautéing an additional 6 minutes, until your mushrooms are lightly browned.
- Enjoy

204) ROASTED ASPARAGUS WITH SESAME SEEDS

Preparation Time: 25 minutes

Servings: 4

Ingredients:

- 1 ½ pounds asparagus, trimmed
- 4 tbsp extra-virgin olive oil
- Sea salt and ground black pepper, to taste
- 1/2 tsp dried oregano
- 1/2 tsp dried basil
- 1 tsp red pepper flakes, crushed
- 4 tbsp sesame seeds
- 2 tbsp fresh chives, roughly chopped

Directions:

- Start by preheating the oven to 400 degrees F. Then, line a baking sheet with parchment paper.
- Toss the asparagus with the olive oil, salt, black pepper, oregano, basil and red pepper flakes. Now, arrange your asparagus in a single layer on the prepared baking sheet.
- Roast your asparagus for approximately 20 minutes.
- Sprinkle sesame seeds over your asparagus and continue to bake an additional 5 minutes or until the asparagus spears are crisp-tender and the sesame seeds are lightly toasted.
- Garnish with fresh chives and serve warm. Enjoy

205) GREEK-STYLE EGGPLANT SKILLET

Preparation Time: 15 minutes

Servings: 4

Ingredients:

- 4 tbsp olive oil
- 1 ½ pounds eggplant, peeled and sliced
- 1 tsp garlic, minced
- 1 tomato, crushed
- Sea salt and ground black pepper, to taste
- 1 tsp cayenne pepper
- 1/2 tsp dried oregano
- 1/4 tsp ground bay leaf
- 2 ounces Kalamata olives, pitted and sliced

Directions:

- Heat the oil in a sauté pan over medium-high flame.
- Then, sauté the eggplant for about 9 minutes or until just tender.
- Add in the remaining ingredients, cover and continue to cook for 2 to 3 minutes more or until thoroughly cooked. Serve warm

206) CAULIFLOWER RICE

Preparation Time: 10 minutes **Servings:** 5

Ingredients:

- 2 medium heads cauliflower, stems and leaves removed
- 4 tbsp extra-virgin olive oil
- 4 garlic cloves, pressed
- 1/2 tsp red pepper flakes, crushed
- Sea salt and ground black pepper, to taste
- 1/4 cup flat-leaf parsley, roughly chopped

Directions:

- Pulse the cauliflower in a food processor with the S-blade until they're broken into "rice".
- Heat the olive oil in a saucepan over medium-high heat. Once hot, cook the garlic until fragrant or about 1 minute.
- Add in the cauliflower rice, red pepper, salt and black pepper and continue sautéing for a further 7 to 8 minutes.
- Taste, adjust the seasonings and garnish with fresh parsley. Enjoy

207) GARLICKY KALE

Preparation Time: 10 minutes **Servings:** 4

Ingredients:

- 4 tbsp olive oil
- 4 cloves garlic, chopped
- 1 ½ pounds fresh kale, tough stems and ribs removed, torn into pieces
- 1 cup vegetable broth
- 1/2 tsp cumin seeds
- 1/2 tsp dried oregano
- 1/2 tsp paprika
- 1 tsp onion powder
- Sea salt and ground black pepper, to taste

Directions:

- In a saucepan, heat the olive oil over a moderately high heat. Now, sauté the garlic for about 1 minute or until aromatic.
- Add in the kale in batches, gradually adding the vegetable broth; stir to promote even cooking.
- Turn the heat to a simmer, add in the spices and let it cook for 5 to 6 minutes, until the kale leaves wilt.
- Serve warm and enjoy

208) ARTICHOKES BRAISED IN LEMON AND OLIVE OIL

Preparation Time: 35 minutes

Servings: 4

Ingredients:

- 1 ½ cups water
- 2 lemons, freshly squeezed
- 2 pounds artichokes, trimmed, tough outer leaves and chokes removed
- 1 handful fresh Italian parsley
- 2 thyme sprigs
- 2 rosemary sprigs
- 2 bay leaves
- 2 garlic cloves, chopped
- 1/3 cup olive oil
- Sea salt and ground black pepper, to taste
- 1/2 tsp red pepper flakes

Directions:

- Fill a bowl with water and add in the lemon juice. Place the cleaned artichokes in the bowl, keeping them completely submerged.
- In another small bowl, thoroughly combine the herbs and garlic. Rub your artichokes with the herb mixture.
- Pour the lemon water and olive oil in a saucepan; add the artichokes to the saucepan. Turn the heat to a simmer and continue to cook, covered, for about 30 minutes until the artichokes are crisp-tender.
- To serve, drizzle the artichokes with cooking juices, season them with the salt, black pepper and red pepper flakes. Enjoy

209) ROSEMARY AND GARLIC ROASTED CARROTS

Preparation Time: 25 minutes

Servings: 4

Ingredients:

- 2 pounds carrots, trimmed and halved lengthwise
- 4 tbsp olive oil
- 2 tbsp champagne vinegar
- 4 cloves garlic, minced
- 2 sprigs rosemary, chopped
- Sea salt and ground black pepper, to taste
- 4 tbsp pine nuts, chopped

Directions:

- Begin by preheating your oven to 400 degrees F.
- Toss the carrots with the olive oil, vinegar, garlic, rosemary, salt and black pepper. Arrange them in a single layer on a parchment-lined roasting sheet.
- Roast the carrots in the preheated oven for about 20 minutes, until fork-tender.
- Garnish the carrots with the pine nuts and serve immediately. Enjoy

LUNCH

The Plant-Based for Athlete

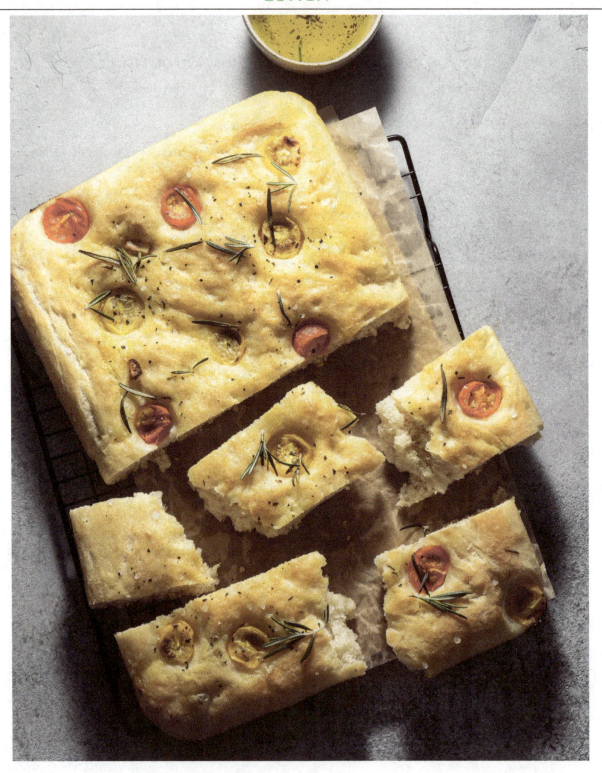

210) MILLET PORRIDGE WITH SULTANAS

Preparation Time: 25 minutes

Servings: 3

Ingredients:

- 1 cup water
- 1 cup coconut milk
- 1 cup millet, rinsed
- 1/4 tsp grated nutmeg
- 1/4 tsp ground cinnamon
- 1 tsp vanilla paste
- 1/4 tsp kosher salt
- 2 tbsp agave syrup
- 4 tbsp sultana raisins

Directions:

- Place the water, milk, millet, nutmeg, cinnamon, vanilla and salt in a saucepan; bring to a boil.
- Turn the heat to a simmer and let it cook for about 20 minutes; fluff the millet with a fork and spoon into individual bowls.
- Serve with agave syrup and sultanas. Enjoy

211) QUINOA PORRIDGE WITH DRIED FIGS

Preparation Time: 25 minutes

Servings: 3

Ingredients:

- 1 cup white quinoa, rinsed
- 2 cups almond milk
- 4 tbsp brown sugar
- A pinch of salt
- 1/4 tsp grated nutmeg
- 1/2 tsp ground cinnamon
- 1/2 tsp vanilla extract
- 1/2 cup dried figs, chopped

Directions:

- Place the quinoa, almond milk, sugar, salt, nutmeg, cinnamon and vanilla extract in a saucepan.
- Bring it to a boil over medium-high heat. Turn the heat to a simmer and let it cook for about 20 minutes; fluff with a fork.
- Divide between three serving bowls and garnish with dried figs. Enjoy

212) BREAD PUDDING WITH RAISINS

Preparation Time: 1 hour

Servings: 4

Ingredients:

- 4 cups day-old bread, cubed
- 1 cup brown sugar
- 4 cups coconut milk
- 1/2 tsp vanilla extract
- 1 tsp ground cinnamon
- 2 tbsp rum
- 1/2 cup raisins

Directions:

- Start by preheating your oven to 360 degrees F. Lightly oil a casserole dish with a nonstick cooking spray.
- Place the cubed bread in the prepared casserole dish.
- In a mixing bowl, thoroughly combine the sugar, milk, vanilla, cinnamon, rum and raisins. Pour the custard evenly over the bread cubes.
- Let it soak for about 15 minutes.
- Bake in the preheated oven for about 45 minutes or until the top is golden and set. Enjoy

213) BULGUR WHEAT SALAD

Preparation Time: 25 minutes **Servings:** 4

Ingredients:

- 1 cup bulgur wheat
- 1 ½ cups vegetable broth
- 1 tsp sea salt
- 1 tsp fresh ginger, minced
- 4 tbsp olive oil
- 1 onion, chopped
- 8 ounces canned garbanzo beans, drained
- 2 large roasted peppers, sliced
- 2 tbsp fresh parsley, roughly chopped

Directions:

- In a deep saucepan, bring the bulgur wheat and vegetable broth to a simmer; let it cook, covered, for 12 to 13 minutes.
- Let it stand for about 10 minutes and fluff with a fork.
- Add the remaining ingredients to the cooked bulgur wheat; serve at room temperature or well-chilled. Enjoy

214) RYE PORRIDGE WITH BLUEBERRY TOPPING

Preparation Time: 15 minutes **Servings:** 3

Ingredients:

- 1 cup rye flakes
- 1 cup water
- 1 cup coconut milk
- 1 cup fresh blueberries
- 1 tbsp coconut oil
- 6 dates, pitted

Directions:

- Add the rye flakes, water and coconut milk to a deep saucepan; bring to a boil over medium-high. Turn the heat to a simmer and let it cook for 5 to 6 minutes.
- In a blender or food processor, puree the blueberries with the coconut oil and dates.
- Ladle into three bowls and garnish with the blueberry topping.
- Enjoy

215) COCONUT SORGHUM PORRIDGE

Preparation Time: 15 minutes **Servings:** 2

Ingredients:

- 1/2 cup sorghum
- 1 cup water
- 1/2 cup coconut milk
- 1/4 tsp grated nutmeg
- 1/4 tsp ground cloves
- 1/2 tsp ground cinnamon
- Kosher salt, to taste
- 2 tbsp agave syrup
- 2 tbsp coconut flakes

Directions:

- Place the sorghum, water, milk, nutmeg, cloves, cinnamon and kosher salt in a saucepan; simmer gently for about 15 minutes.
- Spoon the porridge into serving bowls. Top with agave syrup and coconut flakes. Enjoy

216) MUM'S AROMATIC RICE

Preparation Time: 20 minutes

Servings: 4

Ingredients:

- 3 tbsp olive oil
- 1 tsp garlic, minced
- 1 tsp dried oregano
- 1 tsp dried rosemary
- 1 bay leaf
- 1 ½ cups white rice
- 2 ½ cups vegetable broth
- Sea salt and cayenne pepper, to taste

Directions:

- In a saucepan, heat the olive oil over a moderately high flame. Add in the garlic, oregano, rosemary and bay leaf; sauté for about 1 minute or until aromatic.
- Add in the rice and broth. Bring to a boil; immediately turn the heat to a gentle simmer.
- Cook for about 15 minutes or until all the liquid has absorbed. Fluff the rice with a fork, season with salt and pepper and serve immediately.
- Enjoy

217) EVERYDAY SAVORY GRITS

Preparation Time: 35 minutes

Servings: 4

Ingredients:

- 2 tbsp vegan butter
- 1 sweet onion, chopped
- 1 tsp garlic, minced
- 4 cups water
- 1 cup stone-ground grits
- Sea salt and cayenne pepper, to taste

Directions:

- In a saucepan, melt the vegan butter over medium-high heat. Once hot, cook the onion for about 3 minutes or until tender.
- Add in the garlic and continue to sauté for 30 seconds more or until aromatic; reserve.
- Bring the water to a boil over a moderately high heat. Stir in the grits, salt and pepper. Turn the heat to a simmer, cover and continue to cook, for about 30 minutes or until cooked through.
- Stir in the sautéed mixture and serve warm. Enjoy

218) GREEK-STYLE BARLEY SALAD

Preparation Time: 35 minutes

Servings: 4

Ingredients:

- 1 cup pearl barley
- 2 ¾ cups vegetable broth
- 2 tbsp apple cider vinegar
- 4 tbsp extra-virgin olive oil
- 2 bell peppers, seeded and diced
- 1 shallot, chopped
- 2 ounces sun-dried tomatoes in oil, chopped
- 1/2 green olives, pitted and sliced
- 2 tbsp fresh cilantro, roughly chopped

Directions:

- Bring the barley and broth to a boil over medium-high heat; now, turn the heat to a simmer.
- Continue to simmer for about 30 minutes until all the liquid has absorbed; fluff with a fork.
- Toss the barley with the vinegar, olive oil, peppers, shallots, sun-dried tomatoes and olives; toss to combine well.
- Garnish with fresh cilantro and serve at room temperature or well-chilled. Enjoy

219) SWEET MAIZE MEAL PORRIDGE

Preparation Time: 15 minutes

Servings: 2

Ingredients:

- 2 cups water
- 1/2 cup maize meal
- 1/4 tsp ground allspice
- 1/4 tsp salt
- 2 tbsp brown sugar
- 2 tbsp almond butter

Directions:

- In a saucepan, bring the water to a boil; then, gradually add in the maize meal and turn the heat to a simmer.
- Add in the ground allspice and salt. Let it cook for 10 minutes.
- Add in the brown sugar and almond butter and gently stir to combine. Enjoy

220) DAD'S MILLET MUFFINS

Preparation Time: 20 minutes

Servings: 8

Ingredients:

- 2 cup whole-wheat flour
- 1/2 cup millet
- 2 tsp baking powder
- 1/2 tsp salt
- 1 cup coconut milk
- 1/2 cup coconut oil, melted
- 1/2 cup agave nectar
- 1/2 tsp ground cinnamon
- 1/4 tsp ground cloves
- A pinch of grated nutmeg
- 1/2 cup dried apricots, chopped

Directions:

- Begin by preheating your oven to 400 degrees F. Lightly oil a muffin tin with a nonstick oil.
- In a mixing bowl, mix all dry ingredients. In a separate bowl, mix the wet ingredients. Stir the milk mixture into the flour mixture; mix just until evenly moist and do not overmix your batter.
- Fold in the apricots and scrape the batter into the prepared muffin cups.
- Bake the muffins in the preheated oven for about 15 minutes, or until a tester inserted in the center of your muffin comes out dry and clean.
- Let it stand for 10 minutes on a wire rack before unmolding and serving. Enjoy

221) GINGER BROWN RICE

Preparation Time: 30 minutes

Servings: 4

Ingredients:

- 1 ½ cups brown rice, rinsed
- 2 tbsp olive oil
- 1 (1-inch) piece ginger, peeled and minced
- 1/2 tsp cumin seeds
- Sea salt and ground

Directions:

- Place the brown rice in a saucepan and cover with cold water by 2 inches. Bring to a boil.
- Turn the heat to a simmer and continue to cook for

The Plant-Based for Athlete

- 1 tsp garlic, minced
- black pepper, to taste

- about 30 minutes or until tender.
- ❖ In a sauté pan, heat the olive oil over medium-high heat. Once hot, cook the garlic, ginger and cumin seeds until aromatic.
- ❖ Stir the garlic/ginger mixture into the hot rice; season with salt and pepper and serve immediately

222) CHILI BEAN AND BROWN RICE TORTILLAS

Preparation Time: 50 minutes

Servings: 4

Ingredients:

- ✓ 1 cups brown rice
- ✓ Salt and black pepper to taste
- ✓ 1 tbsp olive oil
- ✓ 1 medium red onion, chopped
- ✓ 1 green bell pepper, diced
- ✓ 2 garlic cloves, minced
- ✓ 1 tbsp chili powder
- ✓ 1 tsp cumin powder
- ✓ 1/8 tsp red chili flakes
- ✓ 1 (15 oz) can black beans, rinsed
- ✓ 4 whole-wheat flour tortillas, warmed
- ✓ 1 cup salsa
- ✓ 1 cup coconut cream for topping
- ✓ 1 cup grated plant-based cheddar

Directions:

- ❖ Add 2 cups of water and brown rice to a medium pot, season with some salt, and cook over medium heat until the water absorbs and the rice is tender, 15 to 20 minutes.
- ❖ Heat the olive oil in a medium skillet over medium heat and sauté the onion, bell pepper, and garlic until softened and fragrant, 3 minutes.
- ❖ Mix in the chili powder, cumin powder, red chili flakes, and season with salt and black pepper. Cook for 1 minute or until the food releases fragrance. Stir in the brown rice, black beans, and allow warming through, 3 minutes. Lay the tortillas on a clean, flat surface and divide the rice mixture in the center of each. Top with the salsa, coconut cream, and plant cheddar cheese. Fold the sides and ends of the tortillas over the filling to secure. Serve immediately

223) CASHEW BUTTERED QUESADILLAS WITH LEAFY GREENS

Preparation Time: 30 minutes

Servings: 4

Ingredients:

- 3 tbsp flax seed powder
- ½ cup cashew cream cheese
- 1 ½ tsp psyllium husk powder
- 1 tbsp coconut flour
- ½ tsp salt
- 1 tbsp cashew butter
- 5 oz grated plant-based cheddar
- 1 oz leafy greens

Directions:

- Preheat oven to 400 F.
- In a bowl, mix flax seed powder with ½ cup water and allow sitting to thicken for 5 minutes. Whisk cashew cream cheese into the vegan "flax egg" until the batter is smooth. In another bowl, combine psyllium husk powder, coconut flour, and salt. Add the flour mixture to the flax egg batter and fold in until incorporated. Allow sitting for a few minutes. Line a baking sheet with wax paper and pour in the mixture. Spread and bake for 5-7 minutes. Slice into 8 pieces. Set aside.
- For the filling, spoon a little cashew butter into a skillet and place a tortilla in the pan. Sprinkle with some plant-based cheddar cheese, leafy greens, and cover with another tortilla. Brown each side of the quesadilla for 1 minute or until the cheese melts. Transfer to a plate. Repeat assembling the quesadillas using the remaining cashew butter. Serve.

224) ASPARAGUS WITH CREAMY PUREE

Preparation Time: 15 minutes

Servings: 4

Ingredients:

- 4 tbsp flax seed powder
- 2 oz plant butter, melted
- 3 oz cashew cream cheese
- ½ cup coconut cream
- Powdered chili pepper to taste
- 1 tbsp olive oil
- ½ lb asparagus, hard stalks removed
- 3 oz plant butter
- Juice of ½ a lemon

Directions:

- In a safe microwave bowl, mix the flax seed powder with ½ cup water and set aside to thicken for 5 minutes. Warm the vegan "flax egg" in the microwave for 1-2 minutes, then pour it into a blender. Add in plant butter, cashew cream cheese, coconut cream, salt, and chili pepper. Puree until smooth.
- Heat olive oil in a saucepan and roast the asparagus until lightly charred. Season with salt and black pepper and set aside. Melt plant butter in a frying pan until nutty and golden brown. Stir in lemon juice and pour the mixture into a sauce cup. Spoon the creamy blend into the center of four serving plates and use the back of the spoon to spread out lightly. Top with the asparagus and drizzle the lemon butter on top. Serve immediately

225) KALE MUSHROOM GALETTE

Preparation Time: 35 minutes

Servings: 4

Ingredients:

- 1 tbsp flax seed powder
- ½ cup grated plant-based mozzarella
- 1 tbsp plant butter
- ½ cup almond flour
- ¼ cup coconut flour
- ½ tsp onion powder
- 1 tsp baking powder
- 3 oz cashew cream cheese, softened
- 1 garlic clove, finely minced
- Salt and black pepper to taste
- 1 cup kale, chopped
- 2 oz cremini mushrooms, sliced
- 2 oz grated plant-based mozzarella
- 1 oz grated plant-based Parmesan
- Olive oil for brushing

Directions:

- Preheat oven to 375 F. Line a baking sheet with parchment paper and grease with cooking spray.
- In a bowl, mix flax seed powder with 3 tbsp water and allow sitting to thicken for 5 minutes. Place a pot over low heat, add in plant-based mozzarella and plant butter, and melt both whiles stirring continuously; remove. Stir in almond and coconut flours, onion powder, baking powder, and ¼ tsp salt. Pour in the vegan "flax egg" and combine until a quite sticky dough forms. Transfer dough to the baking sheet and cover with another parchment paper. Use a rolling pin to flatten into a 12-inch circle.
- After, remove the parchment paper and spread the cashew cream cheese on the dough, leaving about a 2-inch border around the edges. Sprinkle with garlic, salt, and black pepper. Spread kale on top of the cheese, followed by the mushrooms. Sprinkle the plant-based mozzarella and plant-based Parmesan cheese on top. Fold the ends of the crust over the filling and brush with olive oil. Bake until the cheese has melted and the crust golden brown, about 25-30 minutes. Slice and serve with arugula salad

226) FOCACCIA WITH MIXED MUSHROOMS

Preparation Time: 35 minutes

Servings: 4

Ingredients:

- 2 tbsp flax seed powder
- ½ cup tofu mayonnaise
- ¾ cup almond flour
- 1 tbsp psyllium husk powder
- 1 tsp baking powder
- 2 oz mixed mushrooms, sliced
- 1 tbsp plant-based basil pesto
- 2 tbsp olive oil
- Salt and black pepper to taste
- ½ cup coconut cream
- ¾ cup grated plant-based Parmesan

Directions:

- Preheat oven to 350 F.
- Combine flax seed powder with 6 tbsp water and allow sitting to thicken for 5 minutes. Whisk in tofu mayonnaise, almond flour, psyllium husk powder, baking powder, and salt. Allow sitting for 5 minutes. Pour the batter into a baking sheet and spread out with a spatula. Bake for 10 minutes.
- In a bowl, mix mushrooms with pesto, olive oil, salt, and black pepper. Remove the crust from the oven and spread the coconut cream on top. Add the mushroom mixture and plant-based Parmesan cheese. Bake the pizza further until the cheese has melted, 5-10 minutes. Slice and serve with salad

227) SEITAN CAKES WITH BROCCOLI MASH

Preparation Time: 30 minutes

Servings: 4

Ingredients:

- 1 tbsp flax seed powder
- 1 ½ lb crumbled seitan
- ½ white onion
- 2 oz olive oil
- 1 lb broccoli
- 5 oz cold plant butter
- 2 oz grated plant-based Parmesan
- 4 oz plant butter, room temperature
- 2 tbsp lemon juice

Directions:

- Preheat oven to 220 F. In a bowl, mix the flax seed powder with 3 tbsp water and allow sitting to thicken for 5 minutes. When the vegan "flax egg" is ready, add in crumbled seitan, white onion, salt, and pepper. Mix and mold out 6-8 cakes out of the mixture. Melt plant butter in a skillet and fry the patties on both sides until golden brown. Remove onto a wire rack to cool slightly.
- Pour salted water into a pot, bring to a boil, and add in broccoli. Cook until the broccoli is tender but not too soft. Drain and transfer to a bowl. Add in cold plant butter, plant-based Parmesan, salt, and pepper. Puree the ingredients until smooth and creamy. Set aside. Mix the soft plant butter with lemon juice, salt, and pepper in a bowl. Serve the seitan cakes with the broccoli mash and lemon butter

228) SPICY CHEESE WITH TOFU BALLS

Preparation Time: 40 minutes

Servings: 4

Ingredients:

- 1/3 cup tofu mayonnaise
- ¼ cup pickled jalapenos
- 1 tsp paprika powder
- 1 tbsp mustard powder
- 1 pinch cayenne pepper
- 4 oz grated plant-based cheddar
- 1 tbsp flax seed powder
- 2 ½ cup crumbled tofu
- 2 tbsp plant butter

Directions:

- In a bowl, mix tofu mayonnaise, jalapeños, paprika, mustard powder, cayenne powder, and plant-based cheddar cheese; set aside. In another bowl, combine flax seed powder with 3 tbsp water and allow absorbing for 5 minutes. Add the vegan "flax egg" to the cheese mixture, crumbled tofu, salt, and pepper and combine well. Form meatballs out of the mix. Melt plant butter in a skillet and fry the tofu balls until browned. Serve the tofu balls with roasted cauliflower mash

229) QUINOA ANDVEGGIE BURGERS

Preparation Time: 35 minutes

Servings: 4

Ingredients:

- 1 cup quick-cooking quinoa
- 1 tbsp olive oil
- 1 shallot, chopped
- 2 tbsp chopped fresh celery
- 1 garlic clove, minced
- 1 (15 oz) can pinto beans, drained
- 2 tbsp whole-wheat flour
- ¼ cup chopped fresh basil
- 2 tbsp pure maple syrup
- 4 whole-grain hamburger buns, split
- 4 small lettuce leaves for topping
- ½ cup tofu mayonnaise for topping

Directions:

- Cook the quinoa with 2 cups of water in a medium pot until the liquid absorbs, 10 to 15 minutes. Heat the olive oil in a medium skillet over medium heat and sauté the shallot, celery, and garlic until softened and fragrant, 3 minutes.
- Transfer the quinoa and shallot mixture to a medium bowl and add the pinto beans, flour, basil, maple syrup, salt, and black pepper. Mash and mold 4 patties out of the mixture and set aside.
- Heat a grill pan to medium heat and lightly grease with cooking spray. Cook the patties on both sides until light brown, compacted, and cooked through, 10 minutes. Place the patties between the burger buns and top with the lettuce and tofu mayonnaise. Serve

230) BAKED TOFU WITH ROASTED PEPPERS

Preparation Time: 20 minutes

Servings: 4

Ingredients:

- 3 oz cashew cream cheese
- ¾ cup tofu mayonnaise
- 2 oz cucumber, diced
- 1 large tomato, chopped
- 2 tsp dried parsley
- 4 medium orange bell peppers
- 2 ½ cups cubed tofu
- 1 tbsp melted plant butter
- 1 tsp dried basil

Directions:

- Preheat the oven's broiler to 450 F and line a baking sheet with parchment paper. In a salad bowl, combine cashew cream cheese, tofu mayonnaise, cucumber, tomato, salt, pepper, and parsley. Refrigerate.
- Arrange the bell peppers and tofu on the baking sheet, drizzle with melted plant butter, and season with basil, salt, and pepper. Bake for 10-15 minutes or until the peppers have charred lightly and the tofu browned. Remove from the oven and serve with the salad

231) ZOODLE BOLOGNESE

Preparation Time: 45 minutes

Servings: 4

Ingredients:

- 3 oz olive oil
- 1 white onion, chopped
- 1 garlic clove, minced
- 3 oz carrots, chopped
- 3 cups crumbled tofu
- 2 tbsp tomato paste
- 1 ½ cups crushed tomatoes
- Salt and black pepper to taste
- 1 tbsp dried basil
- 1 tbsp vegan Worcestershire sauce
- 2 lb zucchini, spiralized
- 2 tbsp plant butter

Directions:

- Pour olive oil into a saucepan and heat over medium heat. Add in onion, garlic, and carrots and sauté for 3 minutes or until the onions are soft and the carrots caramelized. Pour in tofu, tomato paste, tomatoes, salt, pepper, basil, and Worcestershire sauce. Stir and cook for 15 minutes. Mix in some water if the mixture is too thick and simmer further for 20 minutes. Melt plant butter in a skillet and toss in the zoodles quickly, about 1 minute. Season with salt and black pepper. Divide into serving plates and spoon the Bolognese on top. Serve immediately

232) ZUCCHINI BOATS WITH VEGAN CHEESE

Preparation Time: 40 minutes

Servings: 2

Ingredients:

- 1 medium-sized zucchini
- 4 tbsp plant butter
- 2 garlic cloves, minced
- 1 ½ oz baby kale
- Salt and black pepper to taste
- 2 tbsp unsweetened tomato sauce
- 1 cup grated plant-based mozzarella
- Olive oil for drizzling

Directions:

- Preheat oven to 375 F.
- Use a knife to slice the zucchini in halves and scoop out the pulp with a spoon into a plate. Keep the flesh. Grease a baking sheet with cooking spray and place the zucchini boats on top. Put the plant butter in a skillet and melt over medium heat.
- Sauté the garlic for 1 minute. Add in kale and zucchini pulp. Cook until the kale wilts; season with salt and black pepper. Spoon tomato sauce into the boats and spread to coat the bottom evenly. Then, spoon the kale mixture into the zucchinis and sprinkle with the plant-based mozzarella cheese. Bake for 20-25 minutes. Serve immediately

233) ROASTED BUTTERNUT SQUASH WITH CHIMICHURRI

Preparation Time: 15 minutes

Servings: 4

Ingredients:

- Zest and juice of 1 lemon
- ½ medium red bell pepper, chopped
- 1 jalapeno pepper, chopped
- 1 cup olive oil
- ½ cup chopped fresh parsley
- 2 garlic cloves, minced
- 1 lb butternut squash
- 1 tbsp plant butter, melted
- 3 tbsp toasted pine nuts

Directions:

- In a bowl, add the lemon zest and juice, red bell pepper, jalapeno, olive oil, parsley, garlic, salt, and black pepper. Use an immersion blender to grind the ingredients until your desired consistency is achieved; set aside the chimichurri.
- Slice the butternut squash into rounds and remove the seeds. Drizzle with the plant butter and season with salt and black pepper. Preheat a grill pan over medium heat and cook the squash for 2 minutes on each side or until browned. Remove the squash to serving plates, scatter the pine nuts on top, and serve with the chimichurri and red cabbage salad

234) SWEET AND SPICY BRUSSEL SPROUT STIR-FRY

Preparation Time: 15 minutes

Servings: 4

Ingredients:

- 4 oz plant butter + more to taste
- 4 shallots, chopped
- 1 tbsp apple cider vinegar
- Salt and black pepper to taste
- 1 lb Brussels sprouts
- Hot chili sauce

Directions:

- Put the plant butter in a saucepan and melt over medium heat. Pour in the shallots and sauté for 2 minutes, to caramelize and slightly soften. Add the apple cider vinegar, salt, and black pepper. Stir and reduce the heat to cook the shallots further with continuous stirring, about 5 minutes. Transfer to a plate after.
- Trim the Brussel sprouts and cut in halves. Leave the small ones as wholes. Pour the Brussel sprouts into the saucepan and stir-fry with more plant butter until softened but al dente. Season with salt and black pepper, stir in the onions and hot chili sauce, and heat for a few seconds. Serve immediately

235) BLACK BEAN BURGERS WITH BBQ SAUCE

Preparation Time: 20 minutes

Servings: 4

Ingredients:

- 3 (15 oz) cans black beans, drained
- 2 tbsp whole-wheat flour
- 2 tbsp quick-cooking oats
- ¼ cup chopped fresh basil
- 2 tbsp pure barbecue sauce
- 1 garlic clove, minced
- Salt and black pepper to taste
- 4 whole-grain hamburger buns, split
- For topping:
- Red onion slices
- Tomato slices
- Fresh basil leaves
- Additional barbecue sauce

Directions:

- In a medium bowl, mash the black beans and mix in the flour, oats, basil, barbecue sauce, garlic salt, and black pepper until well combined. Mold 4 patties out of the mixture and set aside.
- Heat a grill pan to medium heat and lightly grease with cooking spray. Cook the bean patties on both sides until light brown and cooked through, 10 minutes. Place the patties between the burger buns and top with the onions, tomatoes, basil, and some barbecue sauce. Serve warm

236) CREAMY BRUSSELS SPROUTS BAKE

Preparation Time: 26 minutes

Servings: 4

Ingredients:

- 3 tbsp plant butter
- 1 cup tempeh, cut into 1-inch cubes
- 1 ½ lb halved Brussels sprouts
- 5 garlic cloves, minced
- 1 ¼ cups coconut cream
- 10 oz grated plant-based mozzarella
- ¼ cup grated plant-based Parmesan
- Salt and black pepper to taste

Directions:

- Preheat oven to 400 F.
- Melt the plant butter in a large skillet over medium heat and fry the tempeh cubes until browned on both sides, about 6 minutes. Remove onto a plate and set aside. Pour the Brussels sprouts and garlic into the skillet and sauté until fragrant.
- Mix in coconut cream and simmer for 4 minutes. Add tempeh cubes and combine well. Pour the sauté into a baking dish, sprinkle with plant-based mozzarella cheese, and plant-based Parmesan cheese. Bake for 10 minutes or until golden brown on top. Serve with tomato salad

237) BASIL PESTO SEITAN PANINI

Preparation Time: 15 minutes + cooling time

Servings: 4

Ingredients:

- For the seitan:
- 2/3 cup basil pesto
- ½ lemon, juiced
- 1 garlic clove, minced
- 1/8 tsp salt
- 1 cup chopped seitan
- For the panini:
- 3 tbsp basil pesto
- 8 thick slices whole-wheat ciabatta
- Olive oil for brushing
- 8 slices plant-based mozzarella
- 1 yellow bell pepper, chopped
- ¼ cup grated plant Parmesan cheese

Directions:

- In a medium bowl, mix the pesto, lemon juice, garlic, and salt. Add the seitan and coat well with the marinade. Cover with plastic wrap and marinate in the refrigerator for 30 minutes.
- Preheat a large skillet over medium heat and remove the seitan from the fridge. Cook the seitan in the skillet until brown and cooked through, 2-3 minutes. Turn the heat off.
- Preheat a panini press to medium heat. In a small bowl, mix the pesto in the inner parts of two slices of bread. On the outer parts, apply some olive oil and place a slice with (the olive oil side down) in the press. Lay 2 slices of plant-based mozzarella cheese on the bread, spoon some seitan on top. Sprinkle with some bell pepper and some plant-based Parmesan cheese. Cover with another bread slice.
- Close the press and grill the bread for 1 to 2 minutes. Flip the bread, and grill further for 1 minute or until the cheese melts and golden brown on both sides. Serve warm

238) SWEET OATMEAL "GRITS"

Preparation Time: 20 minutes

Servings: 4

Ingredients:

- 1 ½ cups steel-cut oats, soaked overnight
- 1 cup almond milk
- 2 cups water
- A pinch of grated nutmeg
- A pinch of ground cloves
- A pinch of sea salt
- 4 tbsp almonds, slivered
- 6 dates, pitted and chopped
- 6 prunes, chopped

Directions:

- In a deep saucepan, bring the steel cut oats, almond milk and water to a boil.
- Add in the nutmeg, cloves and salt. Immediately turn the heat to a simmer, cover and continue to cook for about 15 minutes or until they've softened.
- Then, spoon the grits into four serving bowls; top them with the almonds, dates and prunes.
- Enjoy!

239) FREEKEH BOWL WITH DRIED FIGS

Preparation Time: 35 minutes

Servings: 2

Ingredients:

- 1/2 cup freekeh, soaked for 30 minutes, drained
- 1 1/3 cups almond milk
- 1/4 tsp sea salt
- 1/4 tsp ground cloves
- 1/4 tsp ground cinnamon
- 4 tbsp agave syrup
- 2 ounces dried figs, chopped

Directions:

- Place the freekeh, milk, sea salt, ground cloves and cinnamon in a saucepan. Bring to a boil over medium-high heat.
- Immediately turn the heat to a simmer for 30 to 35 minutes, stirring occasionally to promote even cooking.
- Stir in the agave syrup and figs. Ladle the porridge into individual bowls and serve. Enjoy

240) CORNMEAL PORRIDGE WITH MAPLE SYRUP

Preparation Time: 20 minutes

Servings: 4

Ingredients:

- 2 cups water
- 2 cups almond milk
- 1 cinnamon stick
- 1 vanilla bean
- 1 cup yellow cornmeal
- 1/2 cup maple syrup

Directions:

- In a saucepan, bring the water and almond milk to a boil. Add in the cinnamon stick and vanilla bean.
- Gradually add in the cornmeal, stirring continuously; turn the heat to a simmer. Let it simmer for about 15 minutes.
- Drizzle the maple syrup over the porridge and serve warm. Enjoy

The Plant-Based for Athlete

DINNER

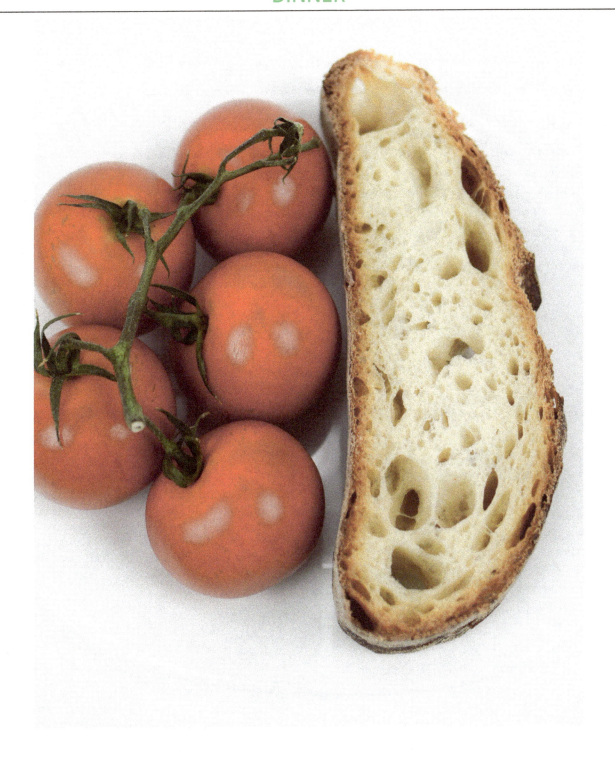

241) MATCHA-INFUSED TOFU RICE

Preparation Time: 35 minutes

Servings: 4

Ingredients:

- 4 matcha tea bags
- 1 ½ cups brown rice
- 2 tbsp canola oil
- 8 oz extra-firm tofu, chopped
- 3 green onions, minced
- 2 cups snow peas, cut diagonally
- 1 tbsp fresh lemon juice
- 1 tsp grated lemon zest
- Salt and black pepper to taste

Directions:

- Boil 3 cups water in a pot. Place in the tea bags and turn the heat off. Let sit for 7 minutes. Discard the bags. Wash the rice and put it into the tea. Cook for 20 minutes over medium heat. Drain and set aside.
- Heat the oil in a skillet over medium heat. Fry the tofu for 5 minutes until golden. Stir in green onions and snow peas and cook for another 3 minutes. Mix in lemon juice and lemon zest. Place the rice in a serving bowl and mix in the tofu mixture. Adjust the seasoning with salt and pepper. Serve right away

242) CHINESE FRIED RICE

Preparation Time: 20 minutes

Servings: 4

Ingredients:

- 2 tbsp canola oil
- 1 onion, chopped
- 1 large carrot, chopped
- 1 head broccoli, cut into florets
- 2 garlic cloves, minced
- 2 tsp grated fresh ginger
- 3 green onions, minced
- 3 ½ cups cooked brown rice
- 1 cup frozen peas, thawed
- 3 tbsp soy sauce
- 2 tsp dry white wine
- 1 tbsp toasted sesame oil

Directions:

- Heat the oil in a skillet over medium heat. Place in onion, carrot, and broccoli, sauté for 5 minutes until tender. Add in garlic, ginger, and green onions and sauté for another 3 minutes. Stir in rice, peas, soy sauce, and white wine and cook for 5 minutes. Add in sesame oil, toss to combine. Serve right away

243) SAVORY SEITAN XAND BELL PEPPER RICE

Preparation Time: 35 minutes **Servings:** 4

Ingredients:
- 2 cups water
- 1 cup long-grain brown rice
- 2 tbsp olive oil
- 1 onion, chopped
- 2 garlic cloves, minced
- 8 oz seitan, chopped
- 1 green bell pepper, chopped
- 1 tsp dried basil
- ½ tsp ground fennel seeds
- ¼ tsp crushed red pepper
- Salt and black pepper to taste

Directions:
- Bring water to a boil in a pot. Place in rice and lower the heat. Simmer for 20 minutes.
- Heat the oil in a skillet over medium heat. Sauté the onion for 3 minutes until translucent. Add in the seitan and bell pepper and cook for another 5 minutes. Stir in basil, fennel, red pepper, salt, and black pepper. Once the rice is ready, remove it to a bowl. Add in seitan mixture and toss to combine. Serve

244) ASPARAGUS AND MUSHROOMS WITH MASHED POTATOES

Preparation Time: 60 minutes **Servings:** 4

Ingredients:
- 5 large portobello mushrooms, stems removed
- 6 potatoes, chopped
- 4 garlic cloves, minced
- 2 tsp olive oil
- ½ cup non-dairy milk
- 2 tbsp nutritional yeast
- Sea salt to taste
- 7 cups asparagus, chopped
- 3 tsp coconut oil
- 2 tbsp nutritional yeast

Directions:
- Place the chopped potatoes in a pot and cover with salted water. Cook for 20 minutes.
- Heat oil in a skillet and sauté garlic for 1 minute. Once the potatoes are ready, drain them and reserve the water. Transfer to a bowl and mash them with some hot water, garlic, milk, yeast, and salt.
- Preheat your grill to medium. Grease the mushrooms with cooking spray and season with salt. Arrange the mushrooms face down and grill for 10 minutes. After, grill the asparagus for about 10 minutes, turning often. Arrange the veggies in a serving platter. Add in the potato mash and serve

245) GREEN PEA AND LEMON COUSCOUS

Preparation Time: 15 minutes **Servings:** 6

Ingredients:
- 1 cup green peas
- 2 ¾ cups vegetable stock
- Juice and zest of 1 lemon
- 2 tbsp chopped fresh thyme
- 1 ½ cups couscous
- ¼ cup chopped fresh parsley

Directions:
- Pour the vegetable stock, lemon juice, thyme, salt, and pepper in a pot. Bring to a boil, then add in green peas and couscous. Turn the heat off and let sit covered for 5 minutes, until the liquid has absorbed. Fluff the couscous using a fork and mix in the lemon and parsley. Serve immediately

246) CHIMICHURRI FUSILI WITH NAVY BEANS

Preparation Time: 25 minutes

Servings: 4

Ingredients:

- 8 oz whole-wheat fusilli
- 1 ½ cups canned navy beans
- ½ cup chimichurri salsa
- 1 cup chopped tomatoes
- 1 red onion, chopped
- ½ cup chopped pitted black olives

Directions:

- n a large pot over medium heat, pour 8 cups of salted water. Bring to a boil and add in the pasta. Cook for 8-10 minutes, drain and let cool. Combine the pasta, beans, and chimichurri in a bowl. Toss to coat. Stir in tomato, red onion, and olives

247) QUINOA AND CHICKPEA POT

Preparation Time: 15 minutes

Servings: 2

Ingredients:

- 2 tsp olive oil
- 1 cup cooked quinoa
- 1 (15-oz) can chickpeas
- 1 bunch arugula chopped
- 1 tbsp soy
- Sea salt and black pepper to taste

Directions:

- Heat the oil in a skillet over medium heat. Stir in quinoa, chickpeas, and arugula and cook for 3-5 minutes until the arugula wilts. Pour in soy sauce, salt, and pepper. Toss to coat. Serve immediately

248) BUCKWHEAT PILAF WITH PINE NUTS

Preparation Time: 25 minutes

Servings: 4

Ingredients:

- 1 cup buckwheat groats
- 2 cups vegetable stock
- ¼ cup pine nuts
- 2 tbsp olive oil
- ½ onion, chopped
- ⅓ cup chopped fresh parsley

Directions:

- Put the groats and vegetable stock in a pot. Bring to a boil, then lower the heat and simmer for 15 minutes. Heat a skillet over medium heat. Place in the pine nuts and toast for 2-3 minutes, shaking often. Heat the oil in the same skillet and sauté the onion for 3 minutes until translucent.
- Once the groats are ready, fluff them using a fork. Mix in pine nuts, onion, and parsley. Sprinkle with salt and pepper. Serve

249)

250) ITALIAN HOLIDAY STUFFING

Preparation Time: 25 minutes

Servings: 4

Ingredients:

- ¼ cup plant butter
- 1 onion, chopped
- 2 celery stalks, sliced
- 1 cup button mushrooms, sliced
- 3 garlic cloves, minced
- ½ cup vegetable broth
- ½ cup raisins
- ½ cup chopped walnuts
- 2 cups cooked quinoa
- 1 tsp Italian seasoning
- Sea salt to taste
- Chopped fresh parsley

Directions:

- In a skillet over medium heat, melt the butter. Sauté the onion, garlic, celery, and mushrooms for 5 minutes until tender, stirring occasionally. Pour in broth, raisins, and walnuts. Bring to a boil, then lower the heat and simmer for 5 minutes. Stir in quinoa, Italian seasoning, and salt. Cook for another 4 minutes. Serve garnished with parsley

251) PRESSURE COOKER GREEN LENTILS

Preparation Time: 30 minutes

Servings: 6

Ingredients:

- 3 tbsp coconut oil
- 2 tbsp curry powder
- 1 tsp ground ginger
- 1 onion, chopped
- 2 garlic cloves, sliced
- 1 cup dried green lentils
- 3 cups water
- Salt and black pepper to taste

Directions:

- Set your IP to Sauté. Add in coconut oil, curry powder, ginger, onion, and garlic. Cook for 3 minutes. Stir in green lentils. Pour in water. Lock the lid and set the time to 10 minutes on High. Once ready, perform a natural pressure release for 10 minutes. Unlock the lid and season with salt and pepper. Serve

252) CHERRY AND PISTACHIO BULGUR

Preparation Time: 45 minutes

Servings: 4

Ingredients:

- 1 tbsp plant butter
- 1 white onion, chopped
- 1 carrot, chopped
- 1 celery stalk, chopped
- 1 cup chopped mushrooms
- 1 ½ cups bulgur
- 4 cups vegetable broth
- 1 cup chopped dried cherries, soaked
- ½ cup chopped pistachios

Directions:

- Preheat oven to 375 F.
- Melt butter in a skillet over medium heat. Sauté the onion, carrot, and celery for 5 minutes until tender. Add in mushrooms and cook for 3 more minutes. Pour in bulgur and broth. Transfer to a casserole and bake covered for 30 minutes. Once ready, uncover and stir in cherries. Top with pistachios to serve

253) MUSHROOM FRIED RICE

Preparation Time: 25 minutes

Servings: 6

Ingredients:

- 2 tbsp sesame oil
- 1 onion, chopped
- 1 carrot, chopped
- 1 cup okra, chopped
- 1 cup sliced shiitake mushrooms
- 2 garlic cloves, minced
- ¼ cup soy sauce
- 1 cups cooked brown rice
- 2 green onions, chopped

Directions:

- Heat the oil in a skillet over medium heat. Place in onion and carrot and cook for 3 minutes. Add in okra and mushrooms, cook for 5-7 minutes. Stir in garlic and cook for 30 seconds. Put in soy sauce and rice. Cook until hot. Add in green onions and stir. Serve warm

254) BEAN AND BROWN RICE WITH ARTICHOKES

Preparation Time: 35 minutes

Servings: 4

Ingredients:

- 2 tbsp olive oil
- 3 garlic cloves, minced
- 1 cup artichokes hearts, chopped
- 1 tsp dried basil
- 1 ½ cups cooked navy beans
- 1 ½ cups long-grain brown rice
- 3 cups vegetable broth
- Salt and black pepper to taste
- 2 ripe grape tomatoes, quartered
- 2 tbsp minced fresh parsley

Directions:

- Heat the oil in a pot over medium heat. Sauté the garlic for 1 minute. Stir in artichokes, basil, navy beans, rice, and broth. Sprinkle with salt and pepper. Lower the heat and simmer for 20-25 minutes. Remove to a bowl and mix in tomatoes and parsley. Using a fork, fluff the rice and serve right away

255) PRESSURE COOKER CELERY AND SPINACH CHICKPEAS

Preparation Time: 50 minutes

Servings: 5

Ingredients:

- 1 cup chickpeas, soaked overnight
- 1 onion, chopped
- 2 garlic cloves, minced
- 1 celery stalk, chopped
- 2 tbsp olive oil
- 3 tsp ground cinnamon
- ½ tsp ground nutmeg
- 1 tbsp coconut oil
- 1 cup spinach, chopped

Directions:

- Place chickpeas in your IP with the onion, garlic, celery, olive oil, 2 cups water, cinnamon, and nutmeg.
- Lock the lid in place; set the time to 30 minutes on High. Once ready, perform a natural pressure release for 10 minutes. Unlock the lid and drain the excess water. Put back the chickpeas and stir in coconut oil and spinach. Set the pot to Sauté and cook for another 5 minutes

256) VEGGIE PAELLA WITH LENTILS

Preparation Time: 50 minutes

Servings: 4

Ingredients:

- 2 tbsp olive oil
- 1 onion, chopped
- 1 green bell pepper, chopped
- 2 garlic cloves, minced
- 1 (14.5-oz) can diced tomatoes
- 1 tbsp capers
- ¼ tsp crushed red pepper
- 1 ½ cups long-grain brown rice
- 3 cups vegetable broth
- 1 ½ cups cooked lentils, drained
- ¼ cup sliced pitted black olives
- 2 tbsp minced fresh parsley

Directions:

- Heat oil in a pot over medium heat and sauté onion, bell pepper, and garlic for 5 minutes. Stir in tomatoes, capers, red pepper, and salt. Cook for 5 minutes. Pour in the rice and broth. Bring to a boil, then lower the heat. Simmer for 20 minutes. Turn the heat off and mix in lentils. Serve garnished with olives and parsley

257) CURRY BEAN WITH ARTICHOKES

Preparation Time: 25 minutes

Servings: 4

Ingredients:

- 1 (14.5-oz) can artichoke hearts, drained and quartered
- 1 tsp olive oil
- 1 small onion, diced
- 2 garlic cloves, minced
- 1 (14.5-oz) can cannellini beans
- 2 tsp curry powder
- ½ tsp ground coriander
- 1 (5.4-oz) can coconut milk
- Salt and black pepper to taste

Directions:

- Heat the oil in a skillet over medium heat. Sauté the onion and garlic for 3 minutes until translucent. Stir in beans, artichoke, curry powder, and coriander. Add in coconut milk. Bring to a boil, then lower the heat and simmer for 10 minutes. Serve

258) ENDIVE SLAW WITH OLIVES

Preparation Time: 10 minutes

Servings: 6

Ingredients:

- 1 lb curly endive, chopped
- ⅓ cup vegan mayonnaise
- ¼ cup rice vinegar
- 2 tbsp vegan yogurt
- 1 tbsp pure date sugar
- 10 black olives for garnish
- ¼ tsp freshly ground black pepper
- ¼ tsp smoked paprika
- ¼ tsp chipotle powder

Directions:

- In a bowl, mix the mayonnaise, vinegar, yogurt, sugar, salt, pepper, paprika, and chipotle powder. Gently add in the curly endive and mix with a wooden spatula to coat. Top with black olives and serve

259) PAPRIKA CAULIFLOWER TACOS

Preparation Time: 40 minutes

Servings: 6

Ingredients:

- 1 head cauliflower, cut into pieces
- 2 tbsp olive oil
- 2 tbsp whole-wheat flour
- 2 tbsp nutritional yeast
- 2 tsp paprika
- 1 tsp cayenne pepper
- Salt to taste
- 1 cups shredded watercress
- 2 cups cherry tomatoes, halved
- 2 carrots, grated
- ½ cup mango salsa
- ½ cup guacamole
- 8 small corn tortillas, warm
- 1 lime, cut into wedges

Directions:

- Preheat oven to 350 F.
- Brush the cauliflower with oil in a bowl. In another bowl, mix the flour, yeast, paprika, cayenne pepper, and salt. Pour into the cauliflower bowl and toss to coat. Spread the cauliflower on a greased baking sheet. Bake for 20-30 minutes.
- In a bowl, combine the watercress, cherry tomatoes, carrots, mango salsa, and guacamole. Once the cauliflower is ready, divide it between the tortillas, add the mango mixture, roll up and serve with lime wedges on the side

SNACKS

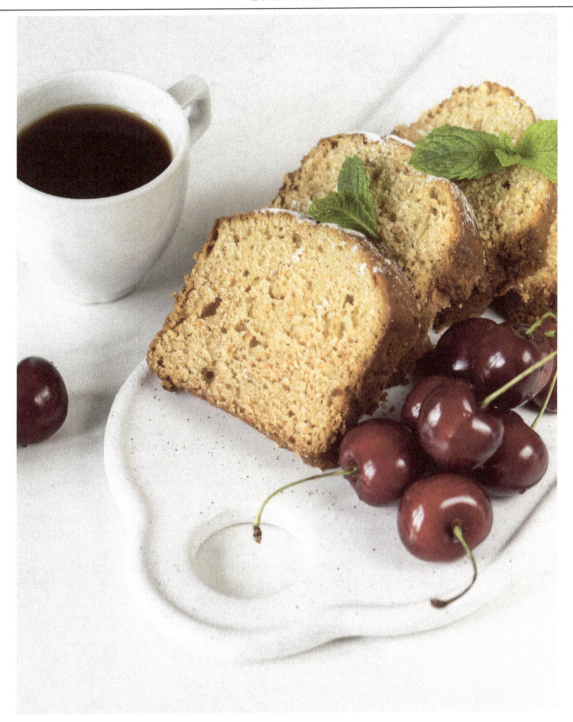

260) FREEKEH SALAD WITH ZA'ATAR

Preparation Time: 35 minutes **Servings:** 4

Ingredients:
- 1 cup freekeh
- 2 ½ cups water
- 1 cup grape tomatoes, halved
- 2 bell peppers, seeded and sliced
- 1 habanero pepper, seeded and sliced
- 1 onion, thinly sliced
- 2 tbsp fresh cilantro, chopped
- 2 tbsp fresh parsley, chopped
- 2 ounces green olives, pitted and sliced
- 1/4 cup extra-virgin olive oil
- 2 tbsp lemon juice
- 1 tsp deli mustard
- 1 tsp za'atar
- Sea salt and ground black pepper, to taste

Directions:
- Place the freekeh and water in a saucepan. Bring to a boil over medium-high heat.
- Immediately turn the heat to a simmer for 30 to 35 minutes, stirring occasionally to promote even cooking. Let it cool completely.
- Toss the cooked freekeh with the remaining ingredients. Toss to combine well.
- Enjoy

261) VEGETABLE AMARANTH SOUP

Preparation Time: 30 minutes **Servings:** 4

Ingredients:
- 2 tbsp olive oil
- 1 small shallot, chopped
- 1 carrot, trimmed and chopped
- 1 parsnip, trimmed and chopped
- 1 cup yellow squash, peeled and chopped
- 1 tsp fennel seeds
- 1 tsp celery seeds
- 1 tsp turmeric powder
- 1 bay laurel
- 1/2 cup amaranth
- 2 cups cream of celery soup
- 2 cups water
- 2 cups collard greens, torn into pieces
- Sea salt and ground black pepper, to taste

Directions:
- In a heavy-bottomed pot, heat the olive oil until sizzling. Once hot, sauté the shallot, carrot, parsnip and squash for 5 minutes or until just tender.
- Then, sauté the fennel seeds, celery seeds, turmeric powder and bay laurel for about 30 seconds, until aromatic.
- Add in the amaranth, soup and water. Turn the heat to a simmer. Cover and let it simmer for 15 to 18 minutes.
- Afterwards, add in the collard greens, season with salt and black pepper and continue to simmer for 5 minutes longer. Enjoy

262) POLENTA WITH MUSHROOMS AND CHICKPEAS

Preparation Time: 25 minutes

Servings: 4

Ingredients:

- 3 cups vegetable broth
- 1 cup yellow cornmeal
- 2 tbsp olive oil
- 1 onion, chopped
- 1 bell pepper, seeded and sliced
- 1 pound Cremini mushrooms, sliced
- 2 garlic cloves, minced
- 1/2 cup dry white wine
- 1/2 cup vegetable broth
- Kosher salt and freshly ground black pepper, to taste
- 1 tsp paprika
- 1 cup canned chickpeas, drained

Directions:

- In a medium saucepan, bring the vegetable broth to a boil over medium-high heat. Now, add in the cornmeal, whisking continuously to prevent lumps.
- Reduce the heat to a simmer. Continue to simmer, whisking periodically, for about 18 minutes, until the mixture has thickened.
- Meanwhile, heat the olive oil in a saucepan over a moderately high heat. Cook the onion and pepper for about 3 minutes or until just tender and fragrant.
- Add in the mushrooms and garlic; continue to sauté, gradually adding the wine and broth, for 4 more minutes or until cooked through. Season with salt, black pepper and paprika. Stir in the chickpeas.
- Spoon the mushroom mixture over your polenta and serve warm. Enjoy

263) TEFF SALAD WITH AVOCADO AND BEANS

Preparation Time: 20 minutes + chilling time

Servings: 2

Ingredients:

- 2 cups water
- 1/2 cup teff grain
- 1 tsp fresh lemon juice
- 3 tbsp vegan mayonnaise
- 1 tsp deli mustard
- 1 small avocado, pitted, peeled and sliced
- 1 small red onion, thinly sliced
- 1 small Persian cucumber, sliced
- 1/2 cup canned kidney beans, drained
- 2 cups baby spinach

Directions:

- In a deep saucepan, bring the water to a boil over high heat. Add in the teff grain and turn the heat to a simmer.
- Continue to cook, covered, for about 20 minutes or until tender. Let it cool completely.
- Add in the remaining ingredients and toss to combine. Serve at room temperature. Enjoy

264) OVERNIGHT OATMEAL WITH WALNUTS

Preparation Time: 5 minutes + chilling time

Servings: 3

Ingredients:

- 1 cup old-fashioned oats
- 3 tbsp chia seeds
- 1 ½ cups coconut milk
- 3 tsp agave syrup
- 1 tsp vanilla extract
- 1/2 tsp ground cinnamon
- 3 tbsp walnuts, chopped
- A pinch of salt
- A pinch of grated nutmeg

Directions:

- Divide the ingredients between three mason jars.
- Cover and shake to combine well. Let them sit overnight in your refrigerator.
- You can add some extra milk before serving. Enjoy

265) COLORFUL SPELT SALAD

Preparation Time: 50 minutes + chilling time

Servings: 4

Ingredients:

- 3 ½ cups water
- 1 cup dry spelt
- 1 cup canned kidney beans, drained
- 1 bell pepper, seeded and diced
- 2 medium tomatoes, diced
- 2 tbsp basil, chopped
- 2 tbsp parsley, chopped
- 2 tbsp mint, chopped
- 1/4 cup extra-virgin olive oil
- 1 tsp deli mustard
- 1 tbsp fresh lime juice
- 1 tbsp white vinegar
- Sea salt and cayenne pepper, to taste

Directions:

- Bring the water to a boil over medium-high heat. Now, add in the spelt, turn the heat to a simmer and continue to cook for approximately 50 minutes, until the spelt is tender. Drain and allow it to cool completely.
- Toss the spelt with the remaining ingredients; toss to combine well and place the salad in your refrigerator until ready to serve.
- Enjoy

266) POWERFUL TEFF BOWL WITH TAHINI SAUCE

Preparation Time: 20 minutes + chilling time

Servings: 4

Ingredients:

- 3 cups water
- 1 cup teff
- 2 garlic cloves, pressed
- 4 tbsp tahini
- 2 tbsp tamari sauce
- 2 tbsp white vinegar
- 1 tsp agave nectar
- 1 tsp deli mustard
- 1 tsp Italian herb mix
- 1 cup canned chickpeas, drained
- 2 cups mixed greens
- 1 cup grape tomatoes, halved
- 1 Italian peppers, seeded and diced

Directions:

- In a deep saucepan, bring the water to a boil over high heat. Add in the teff grain and turn the heat to a simmer.
- Continue to cook, covered, for about 20 minutes or until tender. Let it cool completely and transfer to a salad bowl.
- In the meantime, mix the garlic, tahini, tamari sauce, vinegar, agave nectar, mustard and Italian herb mix; whisk until everything is well incorporated.
- Add the canned chickpeas, mixed greens, tomatoes and peppers to the salad bowl; toss to combine. Dress the salad and toss again. Serve at room temperature. Enjoy

267) POLENTA TOASTS WITH BALSAMIC ONIONS

Preparation Time: 25 minutes + chilling time

Servings: 5

Ingredients:

- 3 cups vegetable broth
- 1 cup yellow cornmeal
- 4 tbsp vegan butter, divided
- 2 tbsp olive oil
- 2 large onions, sliced
- Sea salt and ground black pepper, to taste
- 1 thyme sprig, chopped
- 1 tbsp balsamic vinegar

Directions:

- In a medium saucepan, bring the vegetable broth to a boil over medium-high heat. Now, add in the cornmeal, whisking continuously to prevent lumps.
- Reduce the heat to a simmer. Continue to simmer, whisking periodically, for about 18 minutes, until the mixture has thickened. Stir the vegan butter into the cooked polenta. Spoon the cooked polenta into a lightly greased square baking dish. Cover with the plastic wrap and chill for about 2 hours or until firm.
- Meanwhile, heat the olive oil in a nonstick skillet over a moderately high heat. Cook the onions for about 3 minutes or until just tender and fragrant.
- Stir in the salt, black pepper, thyme and balsamic vinegar and continue to sauté for 1 minute or so; remove from the heat. Cut your polenta into squares. Spritz a nonstick skillet with a cooking spray. Fry the polenta squares for about 5 minutes per side or until golden brown. Top each polenta toast with the balsamic onion and serve. Enjoy

268) FREEKEH PILAF WITH CHICKPEAS

Preparation Time: 40 minutes

Servings: 4

Ingredients:

- 4 tbsp olive oil
- 1 cup shallots, chopped
- 1 celery stalks, chopped
- 1 carrot, chopped
- 1 tsp garlic, minced
- Sea salt and ground black pepper, to taste
- 1 tsp cayenne pepper
- 1 tsp dried basil
- 1 tsp dried oregano
- 1 cup freekeh
- 2 ½ cups water
- 1 cup boiled chickpeas, drained
- 2 tbsp roasted peanuts, roughly chopped
- 2 tbsp fresh mint, roughly chopped

Directions:

- Heat the olive oil in a heavy-bottomed pot over medium-high heat. Once hot, sauté the shallot, celery and carrot for about 3 minutes until just tender.
- Then, add in the garlic and continue to sauté for 30 seconds more or until aromatic. Add in the spices, freekeh and water.
- Turn the heat to a simmer for 30 to 35 minutes, stirring occasionally to promote even cooking. Fold in the boiled chickpeas.
- To serve, spoon into individual bowls and garnish with roasted peanuts and fresh mint. Enjoy

269) GRANDMA'S PILAU WITH GARDEN VEGETABLES

Preparation Time: 45 minutes

Servings: 4

Ingredients:

- 2 tbsp olive oil
- 1 onion, chopped
- 1 carrot, trimmed and grated
- 1 parsnip, trimmed and grated
- 1 celery with leaves, chopped
- 1 tsp garlic, chopped
- 1 cup brown rice
- 2 cups vegetable broth
- 2 tbsp fresh parsley, chopped
- 2 tbsp finely basil, chopped

Directions:

- Heat the olive oil in a saucepan over medium-high heat.
- Once hot, cook the onion, carrot, parsnip and celery for about 3 minutes until just tender. Add in the garlic and continue to sauté for 1 minute or so until aromatic.
- In a lightly oiled casserole dish, place the rice, flowed by the sautéed vegetables and broth.
- Bake, covered, at 375 degrees F for about 40 minutes, stirring after 20 minutes.
- Garnish with fresh parsley and basil and serve warm. Enjoy

The Plant-Based for Athlete

270) EASY BARLEY RISOTTO

Preparation Time: 35 minutes

Servings: 4

Ingredients:

- 2 tbsp vegan butter
- 1 medium onion, chopped
- 1 bell pepper, seeded and chopped
- 2 garlic cloves, minced
- 1 tsp ginger, minced
- 2 cups vegetable broth
- 2 cups water
- 1 cup medium pearl barley
- 1/2 cup white wine
- 2 tbsp fresh chives, chopped

Directions:

- Melt the vegan butter in a saucepan over medium-high heat.
- Once hot, cook the onion and pepper for about 3 minutes until just tender.
- Add in the garlic and ginger and continue to sauté for 2 minutes or until aromatic.
- Add in the vegetable broth, water, barley and wine; cover and continue to simmer for about 30 minutes. Once all the liquid has been absorbed; fluff the barley with a fork.
- Garnish with fresh chives and serve warm. Enjoy

271) TRADITIONAL PORTUGUESE PAPAS

Preparation Time: 35 minutes

Servings: 4

Ingredients:

- 4 cups water
- 2 cups rice milk
- 1 cup grits
- 1/4 tsp grated nutmeg
- 1/4 tsp kosher salt
- 4 tbsp vegan butter
- 1/4 cup maple syrup

Directions:

- Bring the water and milk to a boil over a moderately high heat.
- Stir in the grits, nutmeg and salt. Turn the heat to a simmer, cover and continue to cook, for about 30 minutes or until cooked through.
- Stir in the vegan butter and maple syrup. Enjoy

272) THE BEST MILLET PATTIES EVER

Preparation Time: 40 minutes

Servings: 4

Ingredients:

- 1 cup millet
- 3 cups water
- 2 tbsp olive oil
- 1 onion, finely chopped
- 2 cloves garlic, crushed
- 1 tsp smoked paprika
- 1/2 tsp ground cumin
- Sea salt and ground black pepper, to taste

Directions:

- Bring the millet and water to a boil; turn the heat to a simmer and continue to cook for 30 minutes.
- Fluff your millet with a fork and combine it with the remaining ingredients, except for the oil. Shape the mixture into patties.
- Heat the olive oil in a nonstick skillet over medium-high heat. Fry the patties for 5 minutes per side or until golden-brown and cooked through. Enjoy

The Plant-Based for Athlete

DESSERTS

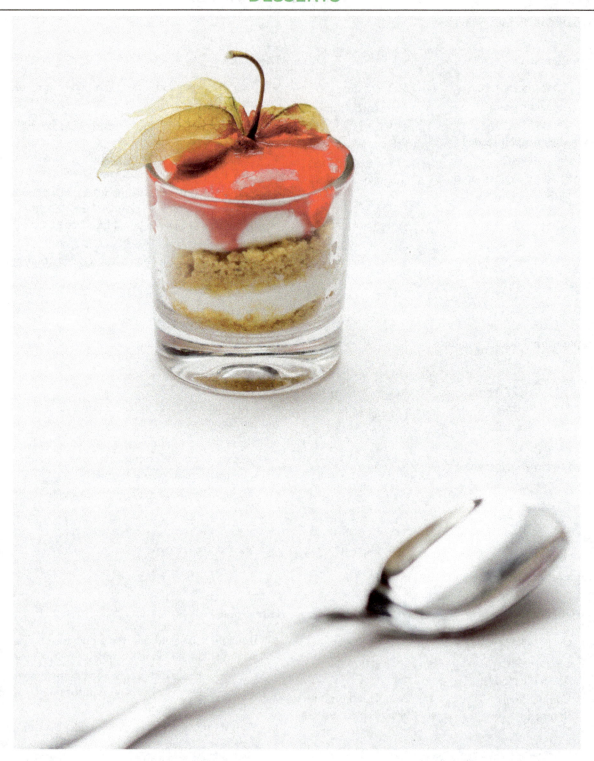

273) AVOCADO TRUFFLES WITH CHOCOLATE COATING

Preparation Time: 5 minutes

Servings: 6

Ingredients:

- 1 ripe avocado, pitted
- ½ tsp vanilla extract
- ½ tsp lemon zest
- 5 oz dairy-free dark chocolate
- 1 tbsp coconut oil
- 1 tbsp unsweetened cocoa powder

Directions:

- Scoop the pulp of the avocado into a bowl and mix with the vanilla using an immersion blender. Stir in the lemon zest and a pinch of salt. Pour the chocolate and coconut oil into a safe microwave bowl and melt in the microwave for 1 minute. Add to the avocado mixture and stir. Allow cooling to firm up a bit. Form balls out of the mix. Roll each ball in the cocoa powder and serve immediately

274) VANILLA BERRY TARTS

Preparation Time: 35 minutes + cooling time

Servings: 4

Ingredients:

- 4 tbsp flaxseed powder
- 1/3 cup whole-wheat flour
- ½ tsp salt
- ¼ cup plant butter, crumbled
- 3 tbsp pure malt syrup
- 6 oz cashew cream
- 6 tbsp pure date sugar
- ¾ tsp vanilla extract
- 1 cup mixed frozen berries

Directions:

- Preheat oven to 350 F and grease mini pie pans with cooking spray. In a bowl, mix flaxseed powder with 12 tbsp water and allow soaking for 5 minutes. In a large bowl, combine flour and salt. Add in butter and whisk until crumbly. Pour in the vegan "flax egg" and malt syrup and mix until smooth dough forms. Flatten the dough on a flat surface, cover with plastic wrap, and refrigerate for 1 hour.
- Dust a working surface with some flour, remove the dough onto the surface, and using a rolling pin, flatten the dough into a 1-inch diameter circle. Use a large cookie cutter, cut out rounds of the dough and fit into the pie pans. Use a knife to trim the edges of the pan. Lay a parchment paper on the dough cups, pour on some baking beans, and bake in the oven until golden brown, 15-20 minutes. Remove the pans from the oven, pour out the baking beans, and allow cooling. In a bowl, mix cashew cream, date sugar, and vanilla extract. Divide the mixture into the tart cups and top with berries. Serve

275) HOMEMADE CHOCOLATES WITH COCONUT AND RAISINS

Preparation Time: 10 minutes + chilling time

Servings: 20

Ingredients:

- 1/2 cup cacao butter, melted
- 1/3 cup peanut butter
- 1/4 cup agave syrup
- A pinch of grated nutmeg
- A pinch of coarse salt
- 1/2 tsp vanilla extract
- 1 cup dried coconut, shredded
- 6 ounces dark chocolate, chopped
- 3 ounces raisins

Directions:

- Thoroughly combine all the ingredients, except for the chocolate, in a mixing bowl.
- Spoon the mixture into molds. Leave to set hard in a cool place.
- Melt the dark chocolate in your microwave. Pour in the melted chocolate until the fillings are covered. Leave to set hard in a cool place.
- Enjoy

276) MOCHA FUDGE

Preparation Time: 1 hour 10 minutes

Servings: 20

Ingredients:

- 1 cup cookies, crushed
- 1/2 cup almond butter
- 1/4 cup agave nectar
- 6 ounces dark chocolate, broken into chunks
- 1 tsp instant coffee
- A pinch of grated nutmeg
- A pinch of salt

Directions:

- Line a large baking sheet with parchment paper.
- Melt the chocolate in your microwave and add in the remaining ingredients; stir to combine well.
- Scrape the batter into a parchment-lined baking sheet. Place it in your freezer for at least 1 hour to set.
- Cut into squares and serve. Enjoy

277) ALMOND AND CHOCOLATE CHIP BARS

Preparation Time: 40 minutes

Servings: 10

Ingredients:

- 1/2 cup almond butter
- 1/4 cup coconut oil, melted
- 1/4 cup agave syrup
- 1 tsp vanilla extract
- 1/4 tsp sea salt
- 1/4 tsp grated nutmeg
- 1/2 tsp ground cinnamon
- 2 cups almond flour
- 1/4 cup flaxseed meal
- 1 cup vegan chocolate, cut into chunks
- 1 1/3 cups almonds, ground
- 2 tbsp cacao powder
- 1/4 cup agave syrup

Directions:

- In a mixing bowl, thoroughly combine the almond butter, coconut oil, 1/4 cup of agave syrup, vanilla, salt, nutmeg and cinnamon.
- Gradually stir in the almond flour and flaxseed meal and stir to combine. Add in the chocolate chunks and stir again.
- In a small mixing bowl, combine the almonds, cacao powder and agave syrup. Now, spread the ganache onto the cake. Freeze for about 30 minutes, cut into bars and serve well chilled. Enjoy

278) ALMOND BUTTER COOKIES

Preparation Time: 45 minutes

Servings: 10

Ingredients:

- 3/4 cup all-purpose flour
- 1/2 tsp baking soda
- 1/4 tsp kosher salt
- 1 flax egg
- 1/4 cup coconut oil, at room temperature
- 2 tbsp almond milk
- 1/2 cup brown sugar
- 1/2 cup almond butter
- 1/2 tsp ground cinnamon
- 1/2 tsp vanilla

Directions:

- In a mixing bowl, combine the flour, baking soda and salt.
- In another bowl, combine the flax egg, coconut oil, almond milk, sugar, almond butter, cinnamon and vanilla. Stir the wet mixture into the dry ingredients and stir until well combined.
- Place the batter in your refrigerator for about 30 minutes. Shape the batter into small cookies and arrange them on a parchment-lined cookie pan.
- Bake in the preheated oven at 350 degrees F for approximately 12 minutes. Transfer the pan to a wire rack to cool at room temperature. Enjoy

279) PEANUT BUTTER OATMEAL BARS

Preparation Time: 25 minutes

Servings: 20

Ingredients:

- 1 cup vegan butter
- 3/4 cup coconut sugar
- 2 tbsp applesauce
- 1 ¾ cups old-fashioned oats
- 1 tsp baking soda
- A pinch of sea salt
- A pinch of grated nutmeg
- 1 tsp pure vanilla extract
- 1 cup oat flour
- 1 cup all-purpose flour

Directions:

- Begin by preheating your oven to 350 degrees F.
- In a mixing bowl, thoroughly combine the dry ingredients. In another bowl, combine the wet ingredients.
- Then, stir the wet mixture into the dry ingredients; mix to combine well.
- Spread the batter mixture in a parchment-lined square baking pan. Bake in the preheated oven for about 20 minutes. Enjoy

280) VANILLA HALVAH FUDGE

Preparation Time: 10 minutes + chilling time

Servings: 16

Ingredients:
- 1/2 cup cocoa butter
- 1/2 cup tahini
- 8 dates, pitted
- 1/4 tsp ground cloves
- A pinch of grated nutmeg
- A pinch coarse salt
- 1 tsp vanilla extract

Directions:
- Line a square baking pan with parchment paper.
- Mix the ingredients until everything is well incorporated.
- Scrape the batter into the parchment-lined pan. Place in your freezer until ready to serve. Enjoy

281) RAW CHOCOLATE MANGO PIE

Preparation Time: 10 minutes + chilling time

Servings: 16

Ingredients:
- Avocado layer:
- 3 ripe avocados, pitted and peeled
- A pinch of sea salt
- A pinch of ground anise
- 1/2 tsp vanilla paste
- 2 tbsp coconut milk
- 5 tbsp agave syrup
- 1/3 cup cocoa powder
- Crema layer:
- 1/3 cup almond butter
- 1/2 cup coconut cream
- 1 medium mango, peeled
- 1/2 coconut flakes
- 2 tbsp agave syrup

Directions:
- In your food processor, blend the avocado layer until smooth and uniform, reserve.
- Then, blend the other layer in a separate bowl. Spoon the layers in a lightly oiled baking pan.
- Transfer the cake to your freezer for about 3 hours. Store in your freezer. Enjoy

282) CHOCOLATE N'ICE CREAM

Preparation Time: 10 minutes

Servings: 1

Ingredients:
- 2 frozen bananas, peeled and sliced
- 2 tbsp coconut milk
- 1 tsp carob powder
- 1 tsp cocoa powder
- A pinch of grated nutmeg
- 1/8 tsp ground cardamom
- 1/8 tsp ground cinnamon
- 1 tbsp chocolate curls

Directions:
- Place all the ingredients in the bowl of your food processor or high-speed blender.
- Blitz the ingredients until creamy or until your desired consistency is achieved.
- Serve immediately or store in your freezer.
- Enjoy

283) RAW RASPBERRY CHEESECAKE

Preparation Time: 15 minutes + chilling time

Servings: 9

Ingredients:
- Crust:
- 2 cups almonds
- 1 cup fresh dates, pitted
- 1/4 tsp ground cinnamon
- Filling:
- 2 cups raw cashews, soaked overnight and drained
- 14 ounces blackberries, frozen
- 1 tbsp fresh lime juice
- 1/4 tsp crystallized ginger
- 1 can coconut cream
- 8 fresh dates, pitted

Directions:
- In your food processor, blend the crust ingredients until the mixture comes together; press the crust into a lightly oiled springform pan.
- Then, blend the filling layer until completely smooth. Spoon the filling onto the crust, creating a flat surface with a spatula.
- Transfer the cake to your freezer for about 3 hours. Store in your freezer.
- Garnish with organic citrus peel. Enjoy

284) MINI LEMON TARTS

Preparation Time: 15 minutes + chilling time

Servings: 9

Ingredients:
- 1 cup cashews
- 1 cup dates, pitted
- 1/2 cup coconut flakes
- 1/2 tsp anise, ground
- 3 lemons, freshly squeezed
- 1 cup coconut cream
- 2 tbsp agave syrup

Directions:
- Brush a muffin tin with a nonstick cooking oil.
- Blend the cashews, dates, coconut and anise in your food processor or a high-speed blender. Press the crust into the peppered muffin tin.
- Then, blend the lemon, coconut cream and agave syrup. Spoon the cream into the muffin tin.
- Store in your freezer. Enjoy

285) COCONUT BLONDIES WITH RAISINS

Preparation Time: 30 minutes

Servings: 9

Ingredients:

- 1 cup coconut flour
- 1 cup all-purpose flour
- 1/2 tsp baking powder
- 1/4 tsp salt
- 1 cup desiccated coconut, unsweetened
- 3/4 cup vegan butter, softened
- 1 ½ cups brown sugar
- 3 tbsp applesauce
- 1/2 tsp vanilla extract
- 1/2 tsp ground anise
- 1 cup raisins, soaked for 15 minutes

Directions:

- Start by preheating your oven to 350 degrees F. Brush a baking pan with a nonstick cooking oil.
- Thoroughly combine the flour, baking powder, salt and coconut. In another bowl, mix the butter, sugar, applesauce, vanilla and anise. Stir the butter mixture into the dry ingredients; stir to combine well.
- Fold in the raisins. Press the batter into the prepared baking pan.
- Bake for approximately 25 minutes or until it is set in the middle. Place the cake on a wire rack to cool slightly.
- Enjoy

286) CHOCOLATE SQUARES

Preparation Time: 1 hour 10 minutes

Servings: 20

Ingredients:

- 1 cup cashew butter
- 1 cup almond butter
- 1/4 cup coconut oil, melted
- 1/4 cup raw cacao powder
- 2 ounces dark chocolate
- 4 tbsp agave syrup
- 1 tsp vanilla paste
- 1/4 tsp ground cinnamon
- 1/4 tsp ground cloves

Directions:

- Process all the ingredients in your blender until uniform and smooth.
- Scrape the batter into a parchment-lined baking sheet. Place it in your freezer for at least 1 hour to set.
- Cut into squares and serve. Enjoy

287) CHOCOLATE AND RAISIN COOKIE BARS

Preparation Time: 40 minutes

Servings: 10

Ingredients:

- 1/2 cup peanut butter, at room temperature
- 1 cup agave syrup
- 1 tsp pure vanilla extract
- 1/4 tsp kosher salt
- 2 cups almond flour
- 1 tsp baking soda
- 1 cup raisins
- 1 cup vegan chocolate, broken into chunks

Directions:

- In a mixing bowl, thoroughly combine the peanut butter, agave syrup, vanilla and salt.
- Gradually stir in the almond flour and baking soda and stir to combine. Add in the raisins and chocolate chunks and stir again.
- Freeze for about 30 minutes and serve well chilled. Enjoy

288) ALMOND GRANOLA BARS

Preparation Time: 25 minutes

Servings: 12

Ingredients:

- 1/2 cup spelt flour
- 1/2 cup oat flour
- 1 cup rolled oats
- 1 tsp baking powder
- 1/2 tsp cinnamon
- 1/2 tsp ground cardamom
- 1/4 tsp freshly grated nutmeg
- 1/8 tsp kosher salt
- 1 cup almond milk
- 3 tbsp agave syrup
- 1/2 cup peanut butter
- 1/2 cup applesauce
- 1/2 tsp pure almond extract
- 1/2 tsp pure vanilla extract
- 1/2 cup almonds, slivered

Directions:

- Begin by preheating your oven to 350 degrees F.
- In a mixing bowl, thoroughly combine the flour, oats, baking powder and spices. In another bowl, combine the wet ingredients.
- Then, stir the wet mixture into the dry ingredients; mix to combine well. Fold in the slivered almonds.
- Scrape the batter mixture into a parchment-lined baking pan. Bake in the preheated oven for about 20 minutes. Let it cool on a wire rack. Cut into bars and enjoy

AUTHOR BIOGRAPHY

THE PLANT-BASED DIET COOKBOOK:

Cook Your Green Passion: 100+ New Tasty Recipes to Try on All Occasions!

THE PLANT-BASED DIET

Cookbook for Beginners

THE PLANT-BASED DIET FOR WOMEN

Simple, Healthy Recipes to Rise Your Everyday Energy and Balance Hormones!

THE PLANT-BASED DIET COOKBOOK FOR ATHLETE

Guide and 100+ Tasty Recipes for a Strong Body and a Healthy Life. Lose Weight and Shape the Body, for Beginners and Experts of All Sports.

THE PLANT-BASED DIET RECIPE BOOK:

2 Books in 1: Easy Beginner's Cookbook with Plant-Based Recipes for Healthy Eating

THE PLANT-BASED DIET FOR BEGINNERS' WOMEN:

2 Books in 1: A Special Guide for Beginners with More than 200 Simple, Healthy Recipes to Rise Your Everyday Energy and Balance Hormones!

THE PLANT-BASED FOR ATHLETE:

2 Books in 1: All You Need to Know About the Plant-Based Diet + More Than 200 Tasty Recipes for a Strong Body and a Healthy Life. Lose Weight and Shape the Body, for Beginners and Experts of All Sports!

THE PLANT-BASED DIET QUICK & EASY:

2 Books in 1: 220+ New Delicious Vegan and Vegetarian Quick & Easy-to-Follow Recipe to Taste!

THE PLANT-BASED DIET FOR MEN:

2 Books in 1: A Game-Changing Approach to Peak Performance! Guide for Beginners: 240+ Quick & Easy, Affordable Recipes that Novice and Busy People Can Do! Reset and Energize Your Body!

THE PLANT-BASED DIET FOR FITNESS:

2 Books in 1: The revolutionary diet book with easy and tasty recipes for healthy and smart people! 240 Fantastic Recipes to Get Fit and Lose Weight!

THE MASTER PLANT-BASED DIET:

3 Books in 1: The Master Guide for Beginners for Vegetarians & Vegans! Try and Taste More than 350 New Recipes and Get to Know About How this Diet Can Help You as Men or Women and Athlete! Special Chapters inside!!!

THE PLANT-BASED DIET FOR BODYBUILDING:

3 Books in 1: 350 Recipes All Vegan & Vegetarian with High-Protein! Beginners Guide to Increase Muscle Mass with Healthy and Whole-Food Vegan Recipes to Fuel Your Workouts!

THE COMPLETE DIET FOR ABSOLUTE BEGINNERS ON PLANT-BASED DIET:

4 Books in 1: Cookbook for Beginners: 470+ Meals to Energize Your Body and Fuel Your Workouts with High-Protein Vegan and Vegetarian Recipes, Healthy and Whole Foods Recipes to Kick-Start a Healthy Eating!

THE PLANT-BASED DIET FOR ONE:

The Revolutionary Recipe Book with Easy and Tasty Recipes for Healthy Lifestyle and Smart People! Lose Rapidly Weight with a Large Choice of 120+ Vegan and Vegetarian Recipes!

THE PLANT-BASED DIET LIKE A RESTAURANT

2 Books in 1: Cook Vegetarian and Vegan Choosing Among Special and Delicious Recipes Like a Chef! Live a Healthy Lifestyle and Lose Rapidly Weight with a Large Choice of 240+ Vegan and Vegetarian Recipes!

THE PLANT-BASED DIET BASICS:

2 Books in 1: All You Need to Know About the Plant-Based Diet + More Than 240 Delicious Vegan and Vegetarian Recipes for Weight Loss and Live Healthy!

THE PLANT-BASED DIET FOR SINGLE:

2 Books in 1: Live a Healthy Lifestyle and Lose Rapidly Weight with a Large Choice of 240+ Vegan and Vegetarian Recipes! Special Guide Included!

THE PLANT-BASED DIET FOR WEIGHT LOSS:

2 Books in 1: Cookbook for Beginners: 240+ Vegetarian and Vegan Recipes to Energize Your Body and Get to Know About How this Diet Can Help to Lose Weight!

THE PLANT-BASED DIET FOR WOMEN OVER 50

3 Books in 1: The Guide and Cookbook for a Simple and Healthy 340+ Recipes to Rise Your Everyday Energy and Balance Hormones!

THE PLANT-BASED DIET FOR MEN OVER 50:

3 Books in 1: A Game-Changing Approach to Peak Performance! 340+ New Delicious Vegan and Vegetarian Quick & Easy-to-Follow Recipe!

THE MASTER EDITION OF PLANT-BASED DIET:

4 Books in 1: A Game-Changing Approach to Peak Performance! 450+ Recipes All Vegan & Vegetarian with High-Protein! Beginners Guide to Live a Healthy Lifestyle! Whole-Food Vegan and Vegetarian Recipes!

CONCLUSIONS

The plant-based diet provides a win-win solution for all those seeking a healthy diet. It protects those suffering from cholesterol and heart disease from saturated animal fats and, on the other hand, saves people from acidic red meat and other animal products that cause toxicity, high blood pressure, etc. This cookbook provides a holistic view of the plant-based diet compromising its basics, known benefits, and all the Dos and Cons. The range of plant-based recipes is covered to meet all everyday needs, including plant-based smoothies, breakfasts, lunch, dinner, and desserts. In addition to these recipes, the book gives a three weak diet plan which allows the best adoption with complete ease and convenience, especially those who weekly prefer to plan their meals.

Thank you for reading this book of the Plant-based diet series!

I hope the recipes could help you to enjoy this diet for delicious meals and reach your goals!

At the beginning of this book, this diet is thought of as a **lifestyle and not as a diet to lose only weight**. A plant-based diet is based on **scientific knowledge to achieve better renal functioning**.

This **Plant-based diet offers almost a flexible approach that adapts to your needs.** The diet allows delicious foods anyway for the whole family, which will take your body and health to the next level!

You deserve to live quietly! If you **no longer** want to live by **becoming crazy,** cooking different dishes for each family member. You will not need to look any further for a **comfortable and healthy diet**.

Thanks very much for reading, and I wish you to achieve your goals and start a new lifestyle!

Audrey Pottery

CPSIA information can be obtained
at www.ICGtesting.com
Printed in the USA
BVHW061925310521
608479BV00007B/1134